Po-Boy Contraband

From Diagnosis Back to Life

by Patrice Melnick

Catalyst Book Press
Livermore, California

Published by Catalyst Book Press
Livermore, California

Summary: Returning home from a stint serving in the Peace Corps in Central Africa, Patrice Melnick learns she is HIV-positive. She decides to live her life to the fullest, appreciating music, food, and literature--and finding love.

The cover art was created by Kelly R. Guidry. His winged figures (as well as other art) are for sale and can be viewed at www.kellyguidry.com.

ISBN 978-0-9802081-4-6
Library of Congress Control Number: 2012936565
June 2012
Printed in the United States of America

To order additional copies of the book, contact Catalyst Book Press
www.catalystbookpress.com
info@catalystbookpress.com

Table of Contents

Forward   7
I. Finding Out
Africa   11
Hospital Moment   19
Babies   21
African Taxi   25
Coins in My Pocket   26
"Blues is the Healer"   30
Music Addict   34
Real Life   37
II. Health, Body and Mortality
Scoring Tickets   40
Oscar   41
Rolling in a Mazda   49
Scars   51
The Opthamologist   54
HIV Survey   57
Rearranging the Furniture   59
Conversation With a Heroin Addict   75
Dating Exam   77
Holding the Wheel   81
III. Dating and Marriage
The Neville Brothers   90
Kissing in the Snow   92
Harmless   101
Zackary   103
Intimacy   107
Support Group   113
Writer's Body   117
NoLove Condoms, Products for our Modern World   123
Gift   125
Thoughts on Writing a Memoir at Forty   128
On Weddings   132

Acknowledgements   145

Po-Boy Contraband

FORWARD

Literary nonfiction is a slippery genre. It is called literary or creative nonfiction to distinguish it from cookbooks and how-to manuscripts. But essayists shape stories, just like fiction writers. While everything you read in this book really happened to me, I may have rearranged time, deleted people because they complicated the story, or zoomed in, like a lens, to focus on a particular person or aspect of the story. If it seems I changed too much, think of this as fiction. If it seems too true to be made up, think of it as nonfiction. Mostly, I hope this book holds your interest and stirs thoughts about your life and the world around you.

This is a memoir of living with HIV and learning to re-evaluate my life. Currently, I live much better than most with this condition. Although these essays are written with hope and humor, do not imagine that the majority of HIV infected population lives so well. The situation I write of is one of privilege with a home, healthcare, family support and relatively little stigma. This is not the case for many others.

While some of the details may echo the experiences of others, I do not pretend to speak for everyone with HIV. Each person's story is unique.

Nevertheless, I hope these writings offer some hope—we all carry burdens in our lives. Through writing, I manage to negotiate life challenges, gain perspective and keep my footing. This book is the outcome of those writings.

Po-Boy Contraband

FINDING OUT

Po-Boy Contraband

Africa

I FIRST BEGAN TO FEEL SICK on the day I went to see the animals. As lions lounged in the brush, the other visitors and I took pictures. After several moments of staring, and clicking cameras, our guide started up the engine again. I remember the surge of nausea as my body absorbed the jolts of the jeep rolling over dirt paths. And I believed I would never again have the opportunity to see wild African animals so close. Although I had lived in Africa for almost two years, I saw very few until I arrived at this remote game preserve. Grey humps of African elephants lumbered along on the forested horizon. Vague sight of swaying trunks, flash of tusks. Flick of ears. Massive, muscular water buffalo stepped through the brush, their delicate noses reaching towards new shoots of grass. Although I did not realize it at the time, I was quite ill. Glimpses of lions and giraffes thrilled me as the sun burned like an infection.

***

I served as a Peace Corps Volunteer from 1985 to 1987 in Bangassou, the Central African Republic. Just a couple months earlier I was thinking of traveling to the wildlife refuge. On that day, I took refuge in my thatched roof house in the spring when wind shook the trees and torrents of rain transformed the neighborhood footpaths into muddy rivers. The air felt fresh and cool and spring mangoes had begun to grow plump. I had found my first two years in the C.A.R. satisfying, so I was considering returning for a 3rd year in the Peace Corps, in Obo, a dry, isolated region near Chad. I felt ready to branch out into new cultural challenges. I enjoyed the isolation in traditional areas where the Zandé people played music and danced the Kpolongo every Saturday night.

Central Africans shook hands, then slid hands gradually apart to snap fingers. Living in Africa felt good to me and I sought as much experience as possible.

***

As spring rains poured, I looked out my window and noticed the water had washed away the red film of dust leaving the leaves of the mango trees brilliant green. I shoved a pan beneath a newly sprouted leak in my roof. In this shadowy house, the *Voice of America* radio station came in clearly in the rain, with dark clouds transmitting radio signals. Paul Simon's new *Graceland* album played "Homeless" with Ladysmith Black Mambazo humming haunting harmonies. My students' English tests screamed to be graded but I remained lost in my daydreams. Through my open door, I saw a boy walk by in the rain selling kerosene. I opened a smelly can of sardines for my hungry cat, Gotabé. School was almost out for summer break, and in the shadows of my house, I began packing for a trip to Ndelé to visit the wildlife preserves. I taught English to children of all ages in a local high school and I longed to break away from my teaching routine, break from the long days of teaching English in hot classrooms packed with 40 to 100 students and then returning home to grade papers. I longed to step onto a bus, one of those open-aired vans packed with tired travelers beneath the roof piled high with luggage, caged chickens and leg-lassoed goats; I longed to board one of those buses to head north to the whispering, wide-open stretches of savannahs to a game preserve near Ndelé. I had always enjoyed moving about independently, to move at my own pace, whether exploring a thatched house neighborhood or following a narrow red dirt path that wound through deep woods. I have always enjoyed daydreaming quietly, slipping into a café alone to enjoy a meal and jot down random thoughts in my journal. I am comfortable with the discomfort of lone travel as I instinctively find my way, in a new town, to a central community bar to ask where to find a safe room to rent for the night. With independence and a bit of arrogance, I wanted to travel solo to the game preserve to see the animals.

***

I climbed out of the road-weary van in Ndelé, my skin coated in red dust, little black bugs biting my ankles. I asked some of the locals where to find Carman, a fellow Peace Corps Volunteer (PCV). It was customary for PCVs to offer lodging to others passing through town. Carmen had stayed with me when she came to Bangassou a few months earlier. When I found her house, she smiled, her broad round face glad for my company, and invited me to stay as long as I wanted. She asked where I was going and how I would get there. I hadn't thought this through. I knew I wanted to see wild animals. I knew I could probably find a ride to the park boundaries. But I had no idea where to stay. Villages probably didn't exist inside the game preserves and certainly not hotels or guest houses. I don't know how I expected to hitchhike through a game preserve, or what I told Carman. Normally, one flies into the region and stays in a resort where tour guides chauffeur the tourists around in open jeeps. Sometimes French, English, or Australian expatriates drive their own Land Rovers into the preserve for the day.

"I wouldn't mind going with you," Carman said in her usual monotone but I sensed enthusiasm.

I couldn't say no. Even my selfishness had limits.

***

I spent a day at Ndelé's police road-barrier, hoping to meet a traveler who was driving through the area I wanted to see. I was prepared to share the cost of gas or pay a small fee. Few vehicles passed through this region, but by the end of the day I had met a kind, youthful French couple, who happened to be game wardens of the national park system. They agreed to give Carmen and me a ride the following day, a ride that brought us several hours into the park. They brought us to their house for the night, a squat, white-washed cement building with a tin roof.

Simone, a large tan woman, shook my hand energetically. She had a round face and straight brown hair pony-tailed beneath her straw hat. Jacques had liquid brown eyes as he stood placidly beside Simone. He shook my hand with slender, surprisingly delicate hands. This memory fades in and out for me. I remember dinner with the couple, but I don't remember what they served. But dining with French ex-patriots—missionaries or international aid workers—was always a treat. Peace Corps volunteers typically ate sardines and stale bread; we probably savored good, imported French cheeses, sausages and wine that night.

***

Carmen and I slept on woven grass mats on the ground, outside of a screened-in guest house. The night air chilled me as Carman and I curled up in our blankets. Inside slept five male French tourists, friends of Simone and Jacques. I lay on my side listening to lions roar in the distance when an ache began to nag inside me. Gas pains or just random discomfort? I curled up against the pain that burrowed into my side. Part of me wanted sympathy or help. I quietly wept. Carman woke up and asked what was wrong, but I didn't know.

"*Ça va?*" one of the Frenchmen asked from inside. Another one woke up, came to the door, and asked if he could help. They invited us to sleep inside on the cement floor.

"*La regle?*" one asked, but I said no, not my period. My period had just passed.

I accepted the muscle relaxant that he offered. I tried to sleep, but continued to hurt throughout the night. I closed my eyes and imagined the bright screams of stars and envisioned the mouths of the lions that roared in the distance. I hoped this pain was nothing serious. I didn't wish to trouble anyone.

In the morning, Carmen and I sat in the sunlit dining room, a room that looked out over a creek where baboons chased each other, bounding over boulders. I did not mention how I felt, hoping the pain would eventually dissolve, but that same morning the French tourists told Simone and Jacques that I was ill. After I confirmed that I felt bad, Jacques radioed the Gounda-Kamboula-Manovo tourist resort in the region, which had plane access. I could be "medevaced" out, if necessary. They decided to drive us from their house to the resort. I wondered how long the trip would last over rutted, dirt roads. The jeep rocked along the rough road like a drunken camel stumbling along in clogs. I clutched my middle. Occasionally, Simone stopped the jeep to point out curl-horned antelope leaping through the brush and giraffes loping in the distance. Sun glare bleached the brittle grass plains. Dark-snouted baboons walked in the dappled shade or sat splay-legged along a riverbank. They flaunted red asses and high-arced tails. The sun glared down upon clusters of antelope. Jacques focused his binoculars, then passed them to me. Tight-muscled antelope loped upon black feet, with horns curving gracefully back. I thought I would never again be able to travel to this remote, lightly-touristed region full of vibrant animals that I had wanted to see all my life.

I had always loved to see animals in the wild, even as a small child camping with my family. "Let's go see the deer, Trecie!" my sisters said, as my parents bundled me up against the frigid Colorado mountain morning at 6:00 a.m when I was six years old. They brought me out of our tent to see a taut-legged mule deer with her spotted fawn that sniffed the breeze and nibbled grass. During my childhood I watched *Wild Kingdom* as Merlin Perkins wrestled with an anaconda, or drugged and tagged a leopard. I am fascinated by the instinctive crouch of a panther, or the nimbleness of a mountain goat. I love to watch bats zig-zag at dusk, radar finely tuned. It is desperate greed I feel when reaching, grabbing for stimulating moments in my life. Even with this alarming pain in my side, I tried to savor the presence of these exotic, graceful animals.

***

At the Gounda-Kamboula-Manovo resort, muscle-shouldered game wardens greeted us with smiles. They had already heard that I wasn't well, and brought Carmen and me to a one-room hut with two beds, a cement floor and thatched roof. They offered to bring me some wild warthog stew to eat, but I didn't feel hungry. I drank part of a coke, and then went to sleep. Later that afternoon, other Central African Republic (CAR) Peace Corps volunteers who were vacationing at the camp visited me. Petite, pig-tailed, brown-eyed Liz, a fellow volunteer and health educator, asked me where I hurt.

"Is it here?" she pointed to the center of her stomach. "Here?" She pointed to one side, then the other. She ruled out a burst appendix. "Maybe an ovary?"

I shrugged.

"Anyone want to go look at animals?" called out the Australian copper-tanned guide that afternoon. I knew I shouldn't go with the mysterious nagging pain that Liz had tried to attribute to one of my organs. But even when I was ill, I could not pass up this lifetime opportunity. I doubted that my condition was life-threatening, and I knew these moments of seeing African animals up close would end too quickly, and could not be duplicated. Six of us piled into an open jeep and bumped along in the hot sun. I cradled my stomach as our guide negotiated the dirt road, wrestling the steering wheel back and forth. Then the guide stopped the jeep, killed the engine and pointed into the brush where a pair of lionesses stared back, cautious, yet calm. One dark-faced cat lay in the shade while the other stood, thick tail swinging gently. Her tawny fur glowed in the glare of the sun and golden eyes gazed apathetically.

A couple hours later, after we returned to the camp, I burrowed into my bed where I slipped in and out of consciousness until the next morning when I boarded a small plane that was owned by the American Baptists who were always willing to help a fellow American in an emergency. The rumble of the engine troubled my insides. The prop turned, then spun and we ascended. I looked out the window down at the dry savannah, hoping to see magnificent, roaming herds of elephants or gazelle like I had seen on *Wild Kingdom* but I saw nothing. The Regional Peace Corps director, Bruce, called me on the plane telephone, though I can't remember what he said. I slept for most of the short flight and awoke as I felt our descent.

Bruce and Abigail waited on the tarmac.

"How are you feeling?" asked Bruce, as he helped me step down from the plane.

"Not so great," I said.

Bruce and Abigail brought me to a private French clinic to see if doctors could diagnose and treat me, or if they would need to fly to the U.S. when the Air France flight arrived in a few days. The U.S. ambassador's wife, who was a nurse, met me at the clinic to assist me. Her name was Rosalyn and she stayed with me when a clinic nurse brought me into an examining room. Several African doctors gathered around me to ask about my symptoms. Then I had to lie down while one of the doctors began to give me a pelvic exam as the others watched. I was glad that Rosalyn had stayed with me. The doctor pushed on my stomach to find out where I hurt, which was everywhere after he began pushing and prodding. The pain cut deeply.

"*Arrete*!" I told him to stop. Rosalyn cringed.

He ended the exam and finally another nurse led me to a single room in which to sleep. I studied the the dimly lit windows and highways of cracks along the walls..

"*Baramo*," I said to the nurse as she straightened the sheets on the bed.

"*Baramo*!" she smiled. She stuck a catheter into the vein on my arm to give me fluids. She and another nurse chatted with me, jumping between French and Sango and speaking these languages made me feel glad because I had positive associations with the C.A.R., and because I was proud of my language abilities. Language helped me to connect to people, and also helped me maintain some independence.

"We'll bring you some food," one of the nurses said.

"No," I said.

"You've got to eat something," she said.

"What kind of food?" I asked. I hadn't eaten for a day, I realized.

"Some meat, potatoes, avocado."

"No."

"You should at least try…"

"No," I couldn't even bear the thought of rich, greasy foods thudding into my sensitive stomach.

She went away.

A nurse brought food and placed the tray in front of me. The tray held a bowl of mussel soup, avocado, bread and butter from an upscale Portuguese restaurant down the road. I ate some of the broth and nibbled the bread. It looked delicious and I wished I had an appetite.

I spent a few days in the clinic, and I enjoyed bantering with the nurses in Sango. I thrived on visits from the Ambassador's kind wife who brought me familiar comfort foods like chicken soup and Jell-O. Later that week, along with a Peace Corps nurse, I boarded an Air France plane to return to the U.S. Towards the front of the plane, I was provided a curtained area with a bed. The nurse gave me a shot of antibiotics mid-flight, as a precaution against what she and the doctors suspected to be an infection. During the flight, when I was awake, I tried to make jokes to make her laugh, but she seemed pensive. I was in denial about my well-being. In Paris, airline workers covered me in a heavy blanket and carried me on a stretcher off the plane. In cold, misty weather, friendly Frenchmen chatted with me as they rolled my hospital bed across the tarmac to an ambulance, and finally to our connecting flight. I hungered to speak French and knew I would miss Africa. I assumed that a doctor would diagnose me, I would be cured and then I would return to taste wild warthog stew and shake hands and snap fingers with Zandé people in Obo. Perhaps I would have another opportunity to visit the preserve.

Hospital Moment

Red African earth was encrusted between my toes, lions roared in my head and a pain gnawed at my side. Sango and French swam in my mind and I had not spoken to my parents in two years, except through letters. I felt cloistered in a sterile room with strangers in pressed, white uniforms walking in and out. A phlebotomist came into my room to draw my blood for the third time since my arrival, as I tried to talk to my parents on the phone.

"You can talk to your mother later," he said. He had a tray of needles and plastic tubes.

"Get out," I said.

He wrapped a rubber strap around my upper arm and slid a needle into my vein as I held the phone in my other hand.

"I'll call back in a little while," I said to my mother. Tears welled up in my eyes once again. The phlebotomist was probably used to emotionally unstable patients.

A sonogram indicated a dermoid cyst on my left ovary, and the doctor said that I needed to go into surgery early the next morning. I later met Dr. Berrigan, who would perform the surgery.

***

"Patrice," a woman's voice said, and I woke up to nausea and a raw soreness in my throat from tubes that reached through my nostrils and down my throat. "You may feel nausea. The tubes will suction your stomach juices into a bag. We don't want you to vomit and strain your stitches," she said.

I saw a motion at the edge of my vision as someone stuck a needle into my hip but I didn't feel it. A greater pain stabbed inside me. I drifted through waves of consciousness, pain, sleep and pain. I remember a Korean nurse who held my hand that night. She said nothing, but the feel of her fingers calmed me. I peered through my post surgery fog and saw my mother holding a bunch of colorful "get well" helium balloons. My panicked parents had flown into town see me. I remember thinking that I should feel happy or appreciative for the cheerful balloons, but I wanted my parents and the bouquet of balloons to float away. I couldn't respond. I don't remember how many days my parents stayed in town. I slept, woke up and saw the faces, heard the voices of one or both of my parents, then I slept again.

Babies

Dr. Berrigan came into my room and said that my right ovary, which had been removed, was the size of a Chicago softball, full of calcium tissue deposits, like hair and teeth. I wondered, *Does a Chicago softball differ from a Philadelphia or Dallas softball?* I was told that women commonly develop harmless dermoid cysts. My ovary had grown large and heavy with cysts until it twisted and became gangrenous. Only later did I grasp the implications of the word "gangrenous," which I associated with dead arms and legs amputated as last resort. I imagined an infection spreading like an oil slick inside of me. I sensed that in the days I rode in jeeps and looked into the eyes of a lion, the situation had become life threatening and the ovary removed just in time.

The doctor described my remaining ovary as fragile, said he didn't dare touch it or it might break off. I imagined it as a wet piece of pink tissue paper ready to tear off and float away into my bodily fluids. I wondered if it would wither like a soft-petaled iris.

"It is *possible* that you can still have children," he said.

The issue of having children hadn't occurred to me.

"Get married, try." He watched me with concern. "Really *try*, and if you can't, see someone, there might be something we can do."

I felt a moment of panic. The doctor showed concern for my reproductive ability, so I felt I should be concerned. But after he left the room I remembered that I didn't want children, ever.

***

When I see a father pacing with an oblong bundle in his arms, I don't have the instinct to look and admire, much less hold the child. I'm more likely to admire a German shepherd puppy or a calico kitten.

"Just wait, you'll change your mind," said family members when I was only a teen. I thought they were probably right since adults were supposed to know more than I. But new offspring in the family was really *their* hope. I never wondered what it was like to have a baby. I don't recall playing with baby dolls and I never owned a Barbie. I remember sensing that I shouldn't want a Barbie doll, too prissy for our feminist-conscious household of the seventies. I only remember playing with troll dolls, passed down from my older sisters. We had about thirty funky-looking, bushy-haired, squat figures and a couple of plastic doll houses that closed up into neat carrying cases with a handle on top. The interior of each house looked cartoonish like a Flintstones cartoon background. In addition to the trolls, stuffed animals, fuzzy bears, cats, snakes, and fantastic creatures covered my bed.

I have wondered, at times, if I have suppressed my urge to have children. Was I in deep denial? Did I really want to become intimate with baby vomit, and slimy strands of saliva? Had I repressed a deep, biological longing? Was this longing overwhelmed by my overly-independent nature?

My biological clock lay broken—I didn't feel a single tick. I could not conjure up even the slightest desire to have a happy lump of baby in my lap, babbling at me as I tried to watch *Austin City Limits* on TV.

***

When I was a teenager, my friend Trinica had cosmetic breast surgery. She said her bras didn't fit right because her breasts were different sizes, so she had the larger one reduced. A day before the surgery, the doctor came in to talk to her. She had to pull up her shirt to expose her breasts. On the breast to be reduced, he quickly drew a web of black circles and lines where the knife would cut.

"Will I be able to breast feed?" she asked the doctor, and he reassured her that she would.

Her inquiry astounded me. Never would I have thought to ask such a question.

At fifteen, she knew she would have children. Subconsciously, I

22

knew I would not. Others might have considered me "young," "less ma-ture." Years later as adults, Trinica had four children, and I had none. So even as teens, we both knew.

It was with reluctance that I entered puberty at 14-years-old. I dreaded the start of my period, and the dark growth of pubic hair. I hoped I would remain flat-chested. I grew huge breasts and wide hips, but re-tained my petite waist. I felt as though I had evolved from a quick little Fiat of a girl into a lumbering Winnebego woman. My breasts flopped awkwardly when I ran. I wanted to hide when men at bus stops gawked at my body; I felt nervous when I rode my bike past construction sites where workers wolf-whistled and cheered as I passed. I felt vulnerable and at times in danger. Friends encouraged me to enjoy the attention by wear-ing tight sweaters but I preferred to hide my figure beneath baggy shirts.

At age 26, perhaps I should have heard my bio-clock ticking in my head, but I only heard my memory-activated internal walkman play-ing Paul Simon's "Diamonds on the Soles of her Shoes," with Ladysmith singing "Sha La La La."

A nurse brought me cranberry juice, as red as menstrual blood. Although I had rejected parts of being female, such as child-bearing, I questioned my womanliness after my ovary was removed.

***

I felt melancholy in the hospital room. With one ovary gone, I tried to contemplate what this meant. Maybe I would never have a child of my own, and though I had never wanted one, I wondered if this made me less feminine. I clung to family voices over the phone. My frail, eighty-eight-year-old grandma told me she made an effort to live so that she could see me again. "Your family is your best friend," she said.

My father had repeated to my grandmother the doctor's advice that I should get married and try to have children.

"That is a very smart doctor!" she said. Her hopes of becoming a great grandmother lay in my womb. She didn't understand her inde-pendent, family-resistant grand-children. At the time neither of my sisters nor my cousins had children. I imagined, one day, gathering with my two sisters and drawing straws. Whoever drew the short one had to make the baby for our parents and grandmother.

I did not want to draw the short straw.

African Taxi

AFTER WALKING AIMLESSLY ALL DAY, feeling lonely in America, I hailed a taxi to go back to the hotel where the Peace Corps volunteers stayed. A yellow cab slowed down and I hopped in the back. As the driver wove through the rush-hour streets, I felt glad to learn that he was Senegalese. He sat tall in the front seat, and had a quick smile as we bantered in French and I felt like I was riding through dirt streets filled with child vendors hawking Fantas and Cokes. He told me he had moved to Washington D.C. two years before to earn money to send to his family back in Senegal. At a traffic light he fished through his glove compartment and pulled out a faded photo of a willowy woman with her green print blouse and long wrap skirt bright against her midnight complexion. She stood surrounded by five children who leaned together and squinted into the sun as they posed. "*Une famille belle,*" I said as I imagined women who carried bowls of mangos on their heads and African guitar music twanged from the huge boom box of a tall skinny boy selling bootleg tapes on a busy street corner; as pedestrians passed the boy, they picked up the rhythm in their hips, carried the beat in their strides. When we arrived at the hotel, I reached into my pocket, hoping I had the right change.

"*Non, ça va!*" the driver waved me on—no charge. Perhaps he shared my nostalgia.

I stepped out of the cab onto the clean sidewalk, and the rain slick streets gleamed.

French syllables clung to my lips as I rode the hotel elevator to my room. I stepped into the bathroom to get ready to take a shower. The vertical cut ran up my abdomen. I studied the threads and red holes and worry stirred inside—part of me was missing.

COINS IN MY POCKET

WHEN I RECEIVED THE PHONE CALL, I had only been home in Dallas, Texas for a week and a half, recovering in the comfort of my parents' home. After two years in Bangassou, I had returned to truly appreciate flush toilets, central air-conditioning, and a refrigerator stocked with roast beef, bagels, cream cheese, and ice cream. In preparation for my third year in the C.A.R, I had bought a couple pair of split skirts, which are modest and functional for bike riding. I had begun recording some of my father's CDs onto cassettes, so I would have a fresh supply of music.

My blood had been drawn before my operation, but I did not know which tests were run. The Peace Corps Administrator I spoke with asked me to come back to D.C. to repeat some blood tests.

"What are the tests for?" I asked her.

"No big deal, we just need to repeat some tests, HIV and some others."

I knew that HIV was the AIDS virus. *I couldn't have heard right.*

"Just come in, we'll sort it out later," she said.

I felt panic, but knew the results must be wrong. I was strong, my appetite huge and my energy level high. Not me.

I made plane reservations and told my parents only that I was returning to Washington D.C. for a follow-up appointment regarding my surgery. They were surprised I had to leave on such short notice. I packed jeans, t-shirts, magazines, a journal, my walkman, cassettes and lots of batteries.

***

I wanted to escape. I had brought with me a tape of Paul Simon's *Graceland.* The lyrical, melodic whirlwind of music spun between the Mississippi Delta, Soweto, Memphis, Lafayette, Senegal, Los Angeles, and New York City. I walked around Washington D.C. wrapped in my private misery. I felt lost between the African guitar whines, and the fast D.C. traffic; between the colorful fabrics in my memory, and D.C. men in polyester power suits. I had fantasies of Paul Simon getting word of a young woman who contracted HIV in Africa, a woman who loved his music. He found out where I lived and took a plane to come visit me at home, the way baseball heroes and basketball stars visit terminally ill, chemo-bald, angel-faced children in hospitals.

***

I sat on a padded, sterile-sheeted examining table in a small, white, florescent-lit room at the Johns Hopkins University Hospital.

"What a shame," said the handsome, dark-haired doctor, "that you contracted this in the prime of your life."

I found no comfort in his words.

I had seen the PBS specials about "AIDS victims," skinny, blue-veined people, bald-headed, walking skeletons, their brains disintegrating as they rolled down linoleum hallways in wheel chairs, or agonized in death beds. Memory loss, fevers, night sweats.

"How long will I live?" I asked the doctor.

"Don't think I can predict that," he said.

"How long?"

"It will be important to eat right, exercise. You may live a long time. You can live a normal life, do anything you want. But you should avoid stress."

I thought of activities that had given me the greatest pleasure in life, working on commercial fishing vessels in Alaska and hiking across the Central African Republic. I wondered if these activities would be considered stressful. I assumed I could not go to the C.A.R. for a third year term.

"Tell me how long."

"You may go three years before you start to have problems," he said, "maybe live five to seven."

I tried to imagine what it would be like to feel the deep sting of open wounds on my body from Karposi's Sarcoma, a condition that I had read about. "Problems" reminded me of the vague language that dentists sometimes used, saying a patient may feel some "discomfort," like a long airline flight or the feel of shoes too small that pinch the big toe or the heel. But the dentist really means that when he starts drilling it will hurt like hell.

"Is mercy killing legal?" I asked.

"No."

"But if you're in pain …" I imagined how I might feel in a few years, as I became ill.

"Morphine kills the pain. How do you feel?" He watched me with very blue eyes beneath dark, thick eyebrows.

I didn't answer.

"Do you feel like killing yourself?"

I shook my head. I could imagine if I was already near death, I might be ready for the pain to end. But I was not ready to go at that moment.

"If you get too depressed," he placed a hand on my shoulder, "if you feel like jumping off a bridge, or out in front of a truck, call me. Will you?"

His statement struck me as odd. I wondered if he might present me with a list of suicide methods to avoid: overdosing on sleeping pills, diving into a swift river, charging into traffic, leaping in front of a train, shooting myself. If I had wanted to die, I would find my HIV diagnosis convenient, delightful. I cried because I wanted to live.

Dr. Doom gave me his card that had several phone numbers so that I could reach him at any time, in case I encountered problems or felt discomfort.

"Did you have unprotected intercourse?"

"Used the pill," I said.

He asked me to detail my sexual activities of the past couple of years. I squirmed. I had a couple of different African boyfriends during my two years in the C.A.R. I didn't want to talk about it. I wondered why he needed to know. For research? Was he gathering statistics? *231 out of 525 AIDS infected patients had swallowed semen, 132 had anal intercourse...* Or was he just curious? His questions made me feel defensive for allowing myself to be exposed to HIV. I was glad to finally escape his office.

"Blues Is The Healer"

I WALKED THE STREETS ALL AFTERNOON, letting the weeping gray sky drench my hair and skin. I listened to the Paul Simon *Graceland* cassette on my walkman. As I passed ornately-gated embassies and quaint Indian import shops, I became lost in the harmonies of Ladysmith Black Mambazo's smooth voices. I thought of the time when I was an undergraduate at the University of Texas. One of my creative writing professors told the class that most of us had never had significant experiences, but he encouraged us to practice writing. I didn't understand until later that he was essentially saying that we were naive kids with nothing important to write about, but if we continued to write, when the time came we would have the skills to handle the human experiences that we encountered. I wondered if the burden of HIV would help me to become a good poet, if I would live long enough to find out. I hoped that the music could hold off hard realities a bit longer. *"Too loo loo, too loo loo."* Joseph Shambalala led the Ladysmith chorus....*"Many dead, tonight it could be you."*

***

During the next week I met with infectious disease specialists, Peace Corps administrators, and psychologists, but I could not concentrate to understand their words. I forgot my English and could barely think. I could only feel.

I remember a Peace Corps health administrator saying that I should get my weight down to where I wanted it, and keep it there. That meant I was too fat, I thought. People handed me pink forms and white forms that I didn't understand how to fill out. The one about disability didn't make sense to me. I thought that meant you had limbs amputated, you limped upon crutches, or couldn't hold a pencil. All my limping was

30

inside. I remember little of what the specialists said to me. I remember concerned brown eyes, blue eyes, green eyes looking into mine for some sign of understanding. *Does the patient comprehend? She just stares.* My eyes ran like undercooked eggs. Through hospital clinic windows, the sun suffocated and my mind went grey.

Paul Simon, Joseph Shabalala and the vibrant chorus of Lady-smith Black Mambazo singers wore bright green and purple tropical prints as they followed me through hospital corridors. I nodded my head to the music while sitting in hospital laboratories waiting for phleboto-mists to draw blood and run more tests. I pulled from my backpack red, dirt-soiled journals that I had written while in Africa and I flipped through the pages, then began new journals. Pain poured onto the pages through stale metaphors and limp images. Recording my thoughts gave me no relief. I could not work through my own numbness. I turned up the walk-man, let the African guitars whine loudly until a woman sitting across from me with hand-drawn eyebrows scowled at me. I turned the music down slightly. But I wanted refuge as I waited for doctors to detail how this disease would destroy my immune system. The words of medical experts spun around me like a foreign language, and sounds blurred into a black noise. Paul Simon's *Graceland* CD had brought a tentative grace into my troubled life.

***

My insides crumpled as I walked in the cold D.C. rain and tried to plan my shortened life. Busy people laughed and hurried by. I feared future years. What would it feel like to have HIV attack my brain? I tuned my Walkman to the Washington D.C. blues station and turned up the volume. Guitar blues and cool voices poured into my ears and the black and white streets gained color and movement and everyone carried rhythm in their walks. I was in a movie with a soundtrack: The newly diagnosed HIV positive woman walks past the stone lions into Georgetown. On a bench John Lee Hooker sits playing his electric guitar and singing. *The blues is a healer*

As Hooker sings, the grey-faced, green-eyed, invisible woman walks through rain-spit puddles. Carlos Santana looms behind John Lee, up in a tree, leaning against a branch as his electric guitar calls out. The woman wanders in and out of bookstores, pausing at the poetry sections as a slow guitar solo whines. Laughing, pony-tailed women brush by, but she doesn't notice. A timbale player at the bottom of the tree thump-thumps heart beats that haunt the damp air. The camera pans the wide-stretched sky of mud-blue smudge clouds, clouds that compose a rhythmic Van Gogh gloom. I felt abnormal among laughing people in colorful cafes. I chewed falafel that tasted like dirt to me. I took in food as a patient takes medicine. I thought about those after-life stories of light coming through tunnels, voices, my life flashing before me. My face felt like the Beatles' stretched out faces on the *Rubber Soul* album cover. Gravity tugged at my thick, grey rubber mask. My face faded in and out among the crowd of people in sunny outfits, beneath beaming umbrellas.

***

In my hotel room, I avoided conversations with other Peace Corps women—they were not meant to be in my movie. I brought the phone into the bathroom to call my mom, but the phone just rang, and then the answering machine picked up. What could I say?

"Hey, Mom, got AIDS in the prime of my life, but don't worry. Be home soon."

I just listened to the answering machine message, then hung up.

I called the Morgans, a family that had lived across the street and whom we had known for about seventeen years. I thought my mom might be there visiting with Rosa Ann, the mother of my friends Laura and Jena. Rosa Ann answered the phone and handed it to my mom.

I faced a wall of white ceramic tile in the shower. "I'm sorry," I said, and the apology echoed back as I told my mother that I had HIV.

"Sorry for what?" she asked.

I couldn't answer. I just felt guilty.

"Do you want us to come up?" she asked.

My throat choked on sobs.

"Trecie?" she repeated.

"I don't know." The cool wall of glacial tiles shined in my eyes.

Knock, Knock, Knock! One of the roommates.

"Just a minute!" I said, trying to steady my voice.

I told my mom, no, I didn't want her to come but I didn't know what I wanted. I felt embarrassed by my explosion of emotions and I wanted to protect my mom from me, from the pain I was causing.

"Talk to her," I heard my mom say, and I could tell she handed the phone to someone else.

"How ya doin'?" I heard Dr. Morgan say. Lester Morgan was a physician, and a calm man. I found his voice and slight drawl comforting

"You know…" he said. "This won't necessarily kill you. No one knows, those doctors, they don't know, you may be just fine."

I didn't believe him, but I liked hearing these words from a doctor, in such contrast to the words of the doctor who had urged me not to jump off a bridge. I slipped these words into my pocket, like a tarnished wheat penny. I fingered the edge of the coin, squeezed the words hard in the palm of my hand. I made a fist around the penny words: *this won't necessarily kill you…those doctors don't know…you may be just fine, just fine, just fine.* The copper words warmed between my fumbling fingers.

Music Addict

I sat on one of the twin beds and my parents sat on the other as they looked through the entertainment section of the newspaper. They had made reservations to fly to D.C. right after I told them of my diagnosis. We were in my parents' hotel room. They asked me what I wanted to do. I wanted to pull into my shell. My mother read aloud about the museum exhibits, the festivals, restaurants, and I felt like the dog in a Far Side cartoon with his master talking to him, but the dog hears, "blah, blah, blah, blah, blah, blah…" The sounds poked my mollusk-soft sides.

"What do you want to do?" My mom began reading aloud the movie listings: "*Tin Men, Raising Arizona, Jaws: The Revenge, Full Metal Jacket, La Bamba, Swimming to Cambodia, Hollywood Shuffle, Surf Nazis Must Die,* …Any of those appeal to you?"

"No, none of that sounds any good." I was a blob on the bed.

Stevie Ray Vaughn appeared across the room and stepped up onto the bedside stand. The movie soundtrack resumed. He launched into a long, whiny, slow-walk electric guitar solo. *"Well, It's floodin' down in Texas."*

Stevie Ray looked great with that black hat dipped down low over his black eyes. His voice howled with stray cat energy.

"We could go to… " my Mom said.

"Nothing," I said. My parents were in the room, Stevie Ray Vaughn was not. He never was. I knew this.

"Would you like to…"

"I don't want to do anything at all." I missed the steady rain.

My parents looked at me for a moment.

"Don't feel like talking. Don't want to do anything. Don't care about anything." I knew that when I went to the movies, I couldn't follow the simplest story. When I ate, I chewed sod. I couldn't absorb colors, or sensations.

"If I could take *this* from you," my father said, "and put it on myself, I would." Dad told me about when I was a newborn and he held me in his arms. He said I was fragile and ill, but Mom and Dad didn't know it. He described the way I squeezed my eyes closed, and I reared my head back. They feared I might be retarded, but it turned out that I had a bladder infection and I responded to pain with the rearing movements, he said. Dad said that he wanted more than anything to protect me, then and at this moment. And I wanted to be protected. My mother wanted the same, but she couldn't bear the pain of silence, she wanted to calm me, and herself, with talk. I realized for the first time that my temperament was more like my father's. I wanted quiet or music. I am my father.

My dad broods. He retreats into his own shell as he reads the *Wall Street Journal,* drives along New Mexico highways and ponders. He speaks little, is more comfortable in the company of quiet. And he likes to turn on the stereo, put on a CD, settle down on the couch, lay his head back and listen to the entire CD.

When my mother feels sad or worried, she busies herself, digging in the garden, or straightening the house. She admits that she is compulsive. She organizes stacks of magazines on the coffee table, rearranges the art objects in her cabinet. She dusts, cleans, shops, chats, and her words whirl into a nervous flurry of activity and conversation to fill the air, to cover over an internal chorus of painful thoughts. My parents didn't know what to *do* with me. I wasn't interested in the movies, museums, or street markets--activities that usually entertained me.

"We don't have to do anything," my father said. "We can just do something quiet."

I realized how much I needed him. The quietness that I had taken for granted most of my life, I needed more than ever.

I remember only flashes of what we did for those few days. I remember bright sunlight, a street fair where I bought an elaborate dangly Indian necklace that I have only worn a few times since. Do the silver jingles remind me of the pain of those days? I don't remember in which restaurants we ate. I didn't want to be with anyone, nor did I want to be alone. Depression bit down onto my heart and I plugged into the relief of my Walkman headphones, like an addict slides a needle in his vein and waits for anxiety to ease. Music didn't ask me to think, didn't try to cheer me, didn't ask me to be positive or focused. The blues kept me company, related to me rather than trying to gloss over my worries or cheer me. It insulated me, soaked me down like rain.

REAL LIFE

A FIVE-FOOT BLOW-UP DINOSAUR stood guard in the corner of Cynthia's living room. I had called up Cynthia and asked if I could stay with her, to get away from the hotel where the other Peace Corps volunteers stayed. She welcomed me to stay in her D.C. apartment for a few days. She lived in a high rise apartment. I had encouraged my parents to return to Dallas, feeling pressured by their attempts to cheer or comfort me. I delayed my return to Dallas, to travel around the D.C. area to visit friends.

I had met Cynthia through one of my Peace Corps friends and we had gone out to lunch once or twice after my operation. She worked as a copy editor for the *Atlantic Monthly*, a magazine that I read avidly, and she took me on a tour of the office. I found comfort in her steady, low voice. I felt awkward telling her about my HIV diagnosis, since I didn't know her well. It seemed to me that people are wary of the emotionally needy, but I told her anyway. Her eyes showed sympathy, but did not seem to grieve. Although I grieved, I did not want the sadness of others to spin me further into my depression.

In some ways I found it easier to talk to someone who did not care about me in the way that a good friend or family member cares. Cynthia told me that she had a gay male friend who also had the virus, and remained healthy. These were the kinds of stories I longed to hear, tales of survivors. Through them, I could perhaps learn to believe in my own survival. I pocketed this thought like another penny and I jingled it against the coin already in my pocket, I jingled the word pennies together, in rhythm, creating a quiet copper tune. At night, as I lay in bed in the spare bedroom, the city lights glistened below like an ocean. While Cynthia was at work all day, I read magazines and listened to music in her sunlit living room. For me, her apartment protected me like a cloud suspended above the city of reality. On my second morning at her house, she telephoned me and suggested we meet at the movies, after work. I wrote down directions on where to meet her.

Cynthia arrived at the theater armed with spicy salami po-boy sandwiches, chips, and drinks, which we smuggled into the theater in a backpack. We watched *Raising Arizona,* an ironic story of a white trash couple stealing a baby, and I was glad for this offbeat movie escape. We sank down into our seats in the dark and the movie's stark scenery reflected in our eyes. We tried to eat the chips quietly, tried not to rattle the bags so we wouldn't get caught and thrown out or have our food confiscated by a dutiful theater usher. I munched the salty chips, and the fizz of the coke cooled my throat. My hunger had returned and we devoured the greasy, spicy salami po-boy contraband, and the outrageous movie about sneaking around and thieving made me laugh; knowing that we were getting away with something made the food taste spicier and richer and although we were escaping in the dark, watching an absurd film, to me this stolen moment tasted like real life.

HEALTH, BODY AND MORTALITY

SCORING TICKETS

IN NEW ORLEANS, I WAS QUEEN of the Ticket Give-Aways! Sometimes
I was the 3rd caller to win tickets from radio stations. I won tickets to
see War at Tipitinas, Tito Puente at the House of Blues. I was surrounded
by brass bands parading down the streets, followed by a serpentine
stream of second line dancers on Sunday afternoons. In the shadows of
19th century brick buildings lingered clusters of old bohemians, young
students, straights and gays, Latinos, Blacks, Whites and occasional
adventurous tourists—there on Frenchman Street on Saturday night
where clubs featured live Jazz, Latin and Reggae music within a two-
block area where I learned to sweat music and dance!

With Radio station phone numbers programmed in my memory
dial, late at night I rang WWOZ, which gave away tickets regularly. With
Gabu on Friday night's "African Journey," I won tickets to Ricardo Lemvo
and Makina Loca—an overdrive orchestra of Afro-Latin, percussive
syncopations. Weekday "Late Night Jazz" tossed me tickets to Mose
Allison. If I had no last-minute available friend to come with me, I went
alone, collected two tickets and then handed one to some astonished
loner standing in line. If solo, I planted myself before the stage, closed
my eyes, soaked in the sounds, and felt like I was in a small living room,
just me and the band. Standing inside the music in tiny, damp, dark
clubs where jazz and funk musicians spun me into a joyous place,
helped me step into my own skin, helped me forget about HIV.

OSCAR

AT MY FIRST UNIVERSITY JOB, I was hired only for a one-year term at a small, private college. The fall semester of my first year was full of turbulent departmental meetings. I felt different from my colleagues in the way I came to the university and the city. Some colleagues had been hired after being flown into New Orleans from distant cities to have a couple days of interviews and finally they were chosen as the best candidates. They may have come to New Orleans for the work and learned to enjoy or tolerate this chaotic, dirty, soulful and often violent city. They tended to be passionate about teaching. I tolerated teaching, but felt passion for New Orleans.

We met in the musty, wood-paneled faculty lounge on the second story. As a new faculty member, I had not yet developed strong opinions about the English Department's curriculum. Sarah, a soft-spoken woman with blond hair and tentative blue eyes, shuffled through her pile of stapled papers. She had brought sample syllabi regarding a literary criticism course that she was hired to develop. The faculty would debate whether the course should be required for all English majors. Some faculty protested the proposed curriculum change. One of the most outspoken was Oscar Lawrence, a tall, lanky man with thinning hair, graying beard, deep wrinkles. He wore khakis and carried a briefcase. He spoke to me with a soft southern accent as we passed in the halls.

After Sarah had distributed the syllabi and discussed the details, Oscar said that to require this course would "be a disservice to our students," and as he spoke, carefully chosen words glinted with double meaning. He pounded his fist on the table for emphasis, then stood up and began to shout. Oscar's eyes glowed with fury, his temples throbbing as his old truck motor voice revved. Sarah silently studied her bare fingernails. I likely would have recoiled from the conflict, as is my nature. Other faculty members' eyes shifted with embarrassment. The department chair suggested we table discussion for a future meeting. Everyone agreed, and I slipped out of the room quickly.

I sensed issues of territory and power, though I did not realize who were allies with whom, and I was unfamiliar with past conflicts, discussions and deceits that had brought them to this stormy moment. In later private conversations, some suggested that as an older faculty member, Oscar might have felt threatened by new approaches to literature as Sarah's course would introduce. I made a mental note to myself not to fight over issues that I didn't care about. There was no need to waste energy, in this precious life, over such struggles.

***

The following weekend, I won tickets to see Kermit Ruffins and the Barbeque Swingers at Vaughn's in the Bywater, an artsy district occupied by tough old folks and hippies who lived in the louver-shuttered old Creole houses. Kermit played every Thursday night at Vaughn's. I arrived around 9:30 p.m. but the band wouldn't start until 11:00 p.m. I felt disoriented inside the tiny, packed barroom. With only about ten tables in the place, people had to stand, as is typical of New Orleans clubs. Clusters of customers crowded the room from the performance area all the way back to the bar and pool room. I saw my friend Richard, a short, fast-talking, dark-eyed man with a sandalwood complexion. He hugged me and spoke briefly but his eyes glanced around the room, searching for other friends. He continued to work his way through the room, embracing each woman he passed. He seemed to know everyone.

I squeezed in between a table and the wall and leaned back to rest my legs. Finally the sounds of drums, piano, trombone and trumpet all merged into an eruption of music that heated the room and I sweated in my celery-hued tank top. People nodded their heads or swayed their upper bodies. One older couple, a skinny man in a gold suit and a rotund woman wearing a tight, shiny fuschia dress and silver heels swung close together in the small floor space before the band—there was no stage. I sipped my coke, shifted my hips from side to side, and finally Kermit, a short, portly man, strode into the room and his gravely voice launched into "If You're a Viper." He flashed a mischievous smile as Eddie Bo's fingers frantically played the keyboard. The performance felt raw, like the worn wood floors, and sound poured through the air like water through collapsed floodgates; my thoughts of Oscar slipped away, and thoughts of papers to be graded melted in the heat of the blasting trumpets. Work concerns dissolved beneath Kermit's playful, gravely voice.

During the break, Kermit barbequed chicken legs on a grill outside on the sidewalk, and served them to fans who slouched against the wall of the building, nursing Abita beers. I stayed until 2:00 a.m., although the music, thick as humidity, hung in the air as I drove away. In New Orleans, clubs can stay open all night long.

***

I came to work only ten minutes before my class on Friday. As I scrambled off to class, my arms full of books, I passed Oscar in the hall and we greeted each other briefly. I hoped that he would never attack me, as he had Sarah.

I felt young and unserious compared to Oscar and other colleagues, most of whom were ten to twenty years older than me. Paranoia grew and I imagined that my playful nature would reveal that I was not a real professor and the department chair would find me undeserving of even this one-year position. I just flitted around in the midnight music clubs. I was no professor, I was a fraud. At one point I was invited to join a creative writing group but I hesitated because most of my material at the time focused on HIV. Revealing myself might put my job even more at risk. Eventually I joined the group where I was careful to write only about other subjects. My condition influenced where I lived, where I worked and my lifestyle. To keep these issues private in writing and conversation made me feel invisible.

***

My department chair, Marta, called me into her office to ask how my classes were going. A mane of wavy brown hair surrounded her narrow face and large brass earrings dangled by her neck as she spoke. She seemed almost motherly with her new faculty members. I told her that my classes seemed fine so far. Then she asked what I thought about the meeting, and I told her it disturbed me. Marta's blue eyes narrowed as she chose her words. She hinted that Oscar didn't like her and that because she had hired me, he would probably dislike me also—like we were high school kids and I was in Marta's clique. Then she told me that she thought that Oscar was anti-Semitic. She warned me to keep up my guard, that he would try to hurt me too, in some way. She specified which department members made up which factions in these verbal faculty sparring matches. Another colleague told me that Oscar had protested against my being hired. When I asked, this same colleague agreed that Oscar might be anti-Semitic. Oscar apparently thought that Sarah was Jewish too, though she wasn't—Marta and I were the only Jewish faculty in the English department.

A couple of days later, on the first cool afternoon of the semester, Oscar stopped me in the hall and asked me to come into his office. I felt a chill, remembering the way he had shouted, and recalling Marta's words. I followed him into his room, a cozy space decorated with a small Asian throw rug. An electric typewriter sat on his desk; in a corner stood a small table with a teapot and a burner, the trappings of a normal person. Oscar sat tall and calm in his leather chair, long legs stretched forward. Wrinkles deepened as he gave his subtle smile. He handed me ten library catalogue cards, and said that each department member was asked to choose ten books that we would like the library to order. I saw no horns growing out of his head and wondered if he saw any growing out of mine. He didn't cackle or grimace; I had never seen him goose step across campus, and his wave in no way resembled a Nazi salute. Hearing his calm, kind voice, I wanted to trust him—he did not seem evil. Oscar asked me to fill out the cards and bring them back in a few weeks. "Thanks," he said, and shook my hand. He did not seem evil.

At the next department meeting, we had just begun to discuss the Literary Criticism proposal when Oscar raised his voice and said, "We would of course all like to require English majors to take each of our specialized courses! Theodore would teach American Literature, Marta would teach Holocaust literature, but that doesn't mean we have the right to require these courses."

Marta glanced at me. She specialized in post-colonial literature—not the Holocaust.

I felt relieved that he had not mentioned me—Oscar did not know my area of interest, and I remained unnoticed.

Finally the department voted in favor of the new curriculum and Oscar stood up in protest. "Well, you've finally ruined me," Oscar said to Marta. "You took me off the hiring committee, you always hire your own kind… and now this!"

I supposed "your own kind" meant Jewish. Oscar then swept his brief case and books under his arm and left the room. The door slammed. The remaining professors looked down silently for a moment. Then we awkwardly continued the discussion.

Later that day, Oscar left xeroxed memos in all of the English department professors' mailboxes, trying to further establish his point, and to criticize the department chair's leadership. As one of the newest faculty members, I was far from tenure and felt vulnerable and invisible.

Oscar fell ill the following year. He began to miss classes and was in the hospital for several weeks. Other professors taught his classes and the next time I saw him he looked thinner and moved with a slow, swift river-crossing motion. Pant legs hung loose like old hide over cow bones, and when he spoke, he almost whispered. Although I distrusted him, having heard his antisemitic-tinged roar, I also felt sorry for him.

I was eventually hired for the Creative Writing position. No one seemed to perceive me as a fake.

***

I answered phones on the AIDS Hotline at the NO/AIDS Task force on Wednesday nights. It was located on Frenchman Street and afterwards

45

I could walk down the street to catch Freddie Omar Con Su Banda at Café Brazil. On one of those evenings at NO/AIDS, I caught sight of Oscar in the office lobby as he hurried in to see a counselor. My first impulse was to say hello, but he didn't see me behind the phone desk. About an hour later, he slipped out. I told my phone partner that I knew the man who had just left.

"That doesn't matter," he said, reminding me of the confidentiality policy.

Other faculty members may have already suspected that Oscar had AIDS. Although he kept his life private, some assumed that he was gay after knowing him for many years. I wondered if Oscar truly disliked me because I was Jewish. Yet I was probably the only person in the department who, like him, had HIV and could have some sense of his sadness and frustration, the pills, the wasting and fears of opportunistic infections that could be terminal. Oscar probably endured the occasional chill of homophobia, a problem I was spared. Yet I still felt alienated with my own secret of HIV.

The following month, at the November departmental meeting, I happened to sit next to Oscar and caught sight of a raw, fleshy, quarter-sized sore on his temple. Later, a colleague told me that he had undergone surgery for a brain tumor. At this meeting, Oscar seemed subdued. He must have been in pain. But I still felt nervous sitting close to him, remembering his previous attacks. Also, I wondered if watching Oscar suffer was like looking through a window into my future. His voice had weakened and he hurled no more clever attacks. No more energy for poison notes.

Oscar continued to spend weeks at a time in the hospital several times and the departmental secretary, at Marta's request, took up a collection for flowers and circulated a "get-well" card for faculty to sign. Some wrote personal notes to Oscar, others just handed over a few dollars. The secretary told us which hospital he was in, but I did not visit him. I was beginning to adjust to my classes, and I was focused on finding balance between overwhelming teaching responsibilities and my social life.

***

During the Thanksgiving holiday, I had lunch with a friend at Jamila's, a new Moroccan restaurant on Maple Street. I happened to glance up towards a sunlit window booth where a haggard old man smiled and waved to me. It took me a moment before I recognized Oscar, with grey stubble on his face and head, hollowed cheeks and sad eyes. He looked glad to see me. He was having lunch with another colleague, an older woman I didn't know well. I walked over to his table and chatted with him briefly, asked how he was feeling, and we talked about the review in the paper about the restaurant. At that moment I regretted not visiting him in the hospital. I was avoiding his anger and avoiding thoughts of my own death etched into his face. At this moment, he looked tired yet tranquil.

***

Oscar had died by the time we returned from the Christmas holiday in January. I vaguely remember a small ceremony in the university chapel. A few people from the English Department read some of Oscar's favorite poems in his honor, though I don't remember which ones. Sarah looked solemn and tense. Others just seemed sad, as if they had forgiven him, and a few loyal female students wept and held hands. I felt only the obligatory sadness that a life had gone, that someone had suffered in the process. I just didn't know how to feel about someone who was so mean, but dead. I felt depressed and afraid for myself as I lingered like an anonymous body in that musical chapel.

One colleague described Oscar years before as warm and delightfully witty. Another colleague, when describing his cruel behavior, would stop and say, "He was very ill…" as if to explain. I wondered if his brain tumor lying against his skull made him mean or if it lay hidden inside him all along, to emerge at the last moments of life. Did the pain make him want to lash out? I wondered if I became ill, would I become mean-spirited? Does illness have effects similar to alcohol, where people become more themselves after a few beers? The red-faced, mean drunks in barrooms shout and raise fists, ready for a brawl. Sappy drunks cling to and kiss acquaintances on the cheek at parties. I wondered which ground swells of emotions would emerge from me. Would I dance and giggle relentlessly? Or would rage bead up on my forehead as I flung my shoe across the room at a stranger with an annoying voice?

This was not a brave time for me. Why didn't I ignore Oscar's hostility and visit him at his home or in the hospital? Would I have told him that I had HIV in hopes of bonding? I acted cowardly and feared that colleagues would find out about me. Years later, I regretted not trying to befriend Oscar. It seemed as if blue poison rivers of anger ran throughout Oscar's body until he tired. And then streams ran clear and calm as the anger dissipated and he died. Although I am not religious, I tried to imagine a heaven where we would meet again. Perhaps Oscar would look peaceful as he did the day we met at Jamila's, sitting by a window, his worry lines muted by the sunlight that warmed the side of his face. In my heaven dream, he would stride through the clouds with a slight bounce in his step. Then he would say something witty and warm and we would dance a waltz and gaze down upon the living who leave poison notes for each other. For a heaven soundtrack, I would prefer a salsa tune while Oscar might prefer a Beethoven symphony, but we would compromise with John Prine's song, "Fish and Whistle," a simple song that carries an ironically upbeat tune: *"We'll whistle and go fishin' the heavens."*

Rolling in a Mazda

When I think about living with HIV, and my experiences with Oscar, I recall an incident that occurred when I was in graduate school at the University of Alaska.

Three fellow students and I packed into an old Mazda and went on a short excursion to Chena Hot Springs, north of Fairbanks. On the return trip, we drove through a snowstorm . I felt drowsy, and considered taking off my seat belt to sleep, but decided against it. I leaned my head against the window and dozed off. I awakened to the slow-motion sensation of the car rolling over, as though we were rolling down the snow covered mountain. I wondered if we'd roll to our deaths. When the car stopped, I was suspended by my seatbelt, upside down. Someone kicked open the door and climbed out. With one hand on the ceiling, I unbuckled my seatbelt and with the other hand I lowered myself to the car ceiling. Each of us climbed out, glad to be alive and unhurt. On looking at the treads in the snow, we realized that when the tires had hit a soft snow bank, the driver overcompensated, trying to steer back onto the road, which caused the car to lean and roll upside down. But at that moment, it felt like we were rolling multiple times. Fortunately we were caravanning with friends in another car and when they looked back to notice us gone, they returned to find us. We all piled into the other car and drove back to Fairbanks.

***

When I think about living with HIV, I have felt like I was in that car, rolling down a mountain. Despite a well-maintained engine and good tires, the road is icy and I wonder to what extent my life is within my control. I feel like Oscar and I rode in the same car, the same storm, snow and sleet hard-tapping against the windshield. The car slides and skids and the front right tire falls into a soft dip and the car begins to roll like a rock tumbler and Oscar and I feel our bodies turn over and over; neither of us deserves to die, neither of us deserves to live, and when the tumbler slows to a stop, Oscar is gone. I breathe deeply and cannot ignore the fact that we rode in the same vehicle; snowstorm gusts sway the trees.

Scars

I KNEW I LIKED ANNETTE WHEN I SAW HER deter a slobbering, stuttering old man who sat next to her and tried to slide his arm around her shoulders.

"Stop it!" she said. "You are not proper, and have no right to show me such disrespect."

"But, I d-d-d-don't mean anythin'... ," he said.

"I won't tolerate it." Annette folded her arms and glared at him.

The man's grin turned down into a frown and he stood up and walked over to a bench in the distance to sit alone. I thought of all the times in cross-cultural situations when I had put up with such behavior because I felt unsure of myself and of the social norms, like the night before when a man at a dance club tried to force his gyrating pelvis against mine. I pulled away and left the club silently. I did not speak up as Annette did.

I met Annette in Bucco Bay, Tobago. She was born in Tobago, but had spent most of her life in England. I arrived in Tobago only a few days before Annette.

"Paradise!" Annette said. "Tobago is paradise." And as she spoke her round, brown face seemed to radiate. We went to the beach together, stretched out on the sand, and listened to the ocean rhythms. A wave rolled in and we both sat up suddenly. Annette was laughing and grabbing at something. "My false breast got away!" she said as she slipped it into her swimsuit top. Then Annette told me that she had breast cancer and one breast was removed. She showed me rigid worms of tissue on the left side of her chest. "Do you want to feel it?" she asked as she pulled the prosthetic breast out and offered it in the palm of her hand. Her candidness startled me, but I didn't dare refuse. I admired her honest power. The false breast felt rubbery, like a small water balloon, but slicker, heavier and more firm.

I showed Annette a slightly angled, whitish, 5-inch scar a few inches below my right knee. At 17, a car hit me as I rode my bicycle and the scar still remains. Small dots ran along each side of the ridge where the skin was once sewn together. Annette nodded. On my left knee, a 3-inch long white scar from an incident, while floating in inner tubes down the Gruene River in Texas. I fell out of my inner-tube and cut my knee on a sharp rock. And I showed her dime-sized dark spots on my legs from infected mosquito bites I acquired during my Peace Corps years, trying to reciprocate her openness. I thought about telling her that I had HIV, but I withheld.

Annette and I talked about men. She had been married twice, and wished she could have a baby with her second husband but she'd had a hysterectomy. We sat on the shore and squealed as the cool rush of ocean ran over our legs. I spread sunscreen on my body, where ever I could reach. She rubbed some lotion in the middle of my back. Though she was brown, and I was white, we both stretched out hoping for more color. Annette refused my offer of sun block—said she was too pale after all those years in England.

I showed Annette my largest scar, the hard white line that stretched from the edge of my bikini bottom up to my navel. I told her about coming from Africa, flying to Washington D.C., rushed to the hospital to be operated on to remove the gangrenous ovary "the size of a Chicago softball." She asked me if I wanted children. I admitted I probably couldn't have them but didn't specify why, citing vague health problems. She said I might later regret not having them.

Flocks of bright green parrots screeched overhead. Annette looked at me sympathetically. I couldn't say anymore.

Years later, I kept thinking about the things I didn't tell her. I am not sure why I didn't reveal my HIV status except that at the time I did not tell new acquaintances. Perhaps I feared a negative response, or I feared talking about it would unlock my own vault of emotion, making her uncomfortable. But I know for sure that if I could be there again, stretched out on the beach next to Annette, I would have told her that I had HIV.

Annette seemed unconcerned about what others thought about her. She must have understood that everyone has their own problems. She seemed to know that her life was her own, the imperfections, the sadness, the joy; and she swam through the water, driven by a propulsion of truth, and revealing. I recalled the times that I had revealed my HIV status and the world around me did not collapse. Friends did not recoil and we grew closer, savoring the precious silk of life. I have continued to think of Annette when I meet others and want to speak and live openly.

The Ophthalmologist

I WENT TO AN OPHTHALMOLOGIST to be sure that a recent bout with shingles had not damaged my eye. I dutifully filled out the paperwork and checked off boxes regarding medical history. I paused for only a moment as I checked off the HIV box. It was a cold March day in Fairbanks, Alaska and my parka lay wadded up on the chair beside me as I waited.

"This might sting a moment," said the bald-headed, ruddy-faced doctor as he put drops into my eyes. "Not too uncommon for AIDS patients to get shingles."

I am not an AIDS patient, I thought, *I have HIV*. In my mind, having HIV meant I had not yet become terminally ill. Shingles was not one of the Opportunistic Infections (OIs). I had heard of Pneumocystis Pneumonia or Karposi's Sarcoma, extremely rare diseases. Regular people got shingles. The healthy, portly nurse at the hospital told me that she had shingles once. This meant that normal people got them, I was not different, not yet. It was not an opportunistic Infection therefore I did not have AIDS—I needed to believe this. I clung to the HIV definition. "AIDS patient" meant I belonged in a hospice, needed constant medical care, was in and out of hospitals; AIDS meant it was too late for me. My face was warm, my hands clammy. "I think of myself as having HIV," I said.

"Uh huh," the doctor nodded. "So, you got HIV from a blood transfusion?" he asked.

"No." My vision grew blurry from the drops.

"Wait just a minute for your eyes to dilate," the doctor said. "So, not from a blood transfusion?"

"No." I wondered why he asked how I had been infected and why he assumed blood transfusion. Did blood transfusion seem the most

54

likely way in which a woman would become infected? Did he think I seemed like a "nice girl" and therefore couldn't have gotten HIV from sex or sharing needles? I hoped that he was not trying to figure me into his assessment of "guilt" or "innocence." I did not feel more or less guilty than anyone else.

"I'll be right back," the doctor said as he walked out the door. I sat in the blue-grey room until he returned and shut off the lights. He shone a light into each eye. "So where did you get it from?" His tone was friendly, casual. Perhaps he was just trying to make conversation.

"From sex," I said. "Sex with a man." I hoped the questions would end.

He projected onto the wall an eye-chart. I think I read most of the letters right.

"That's fine," he said as he switched on the lights.

I could hear the soft buzz of a flickering light bulb.

"Do you know from who?" he asked.

I couldn't figure out how to make the doctor stop asking questions without being rude. He seemed nosy, like a man that peers through the midnight, bedroom window of his neighbor's house. Was he trying to figure out if I was "guilty" or a "victim?"

"Got it in the Central African Republic," I said, "in the Peace Corps." I hoped he'd be satisfied.

"Not too much scarring," the doctor said as he scribbled something into my chart. "Vision seems fine. Was it from a white man or a black man?"

My stomach tightened into a fist. White or Black? Good or bad? My heart raced. I felt like the doctor had shifted me from the "blood-transfusion—victim" box to the "sex—guilt" box and now he was trying to figure out whether to toss me from the "sex-with-white-man" box down into the "sex-with-black-man" box.

Was he trying to imagine scenes, as though watching a movie in his mind? Was he trying to figure out if this was *Sleepless in Seattle* or *Jungle Fever*? *Love Story* or *Guess Who's Coming to Dinner*? *When Harry Met*

Sally or *Zebra Head*? I wondered who would play me in the love scenes? Not Julia Roberts or Meg Ryan. Too glamorous. Maybe Janeane Garafolo or Francis McDermott, down-to-earth. But the doctor was wondering who would play the male lead. Johnny Depp or Denzel Washington? Brad Pitt or Wesley Snipes? John Cussack or Samuel L. Jackson? Would there be full-frontal nudity? Surely the obligatory flash of breasts. Would the actress do her own love scenes or have a double? Would there be male frontal nudity, a-la-Harvey-Keitel-The Piano? But would nudity harm or help the ratings? Would the production inch into soft porn? The doctor wanted the details, he wanted to *see* the story, people want to *see* the story—the public wants details, bare flesh! This was no longer a medical situation, a virus, a patient; this was skin, this was racy, this was race.

But it was also about boxes, the innocent-victim box versus the got-what-she-deserved box. And I seemed like a nice girl, I was going to graduate school, my clothes were clean, my skin was pale, I spoke standard English and I had a pretty smile in the right light, if you don't look too close.

I envisioned some of my African friends: Mariam Hamat ran vividly printed meters of fabric between her fingers; Awa's slender, coffee-toned hands braided her sister's hair. The upbeat guitar solos of the Central African band *Makembe* played in my head, vocal harmonies sang in my veins.

The doctor's blue eyes scanned my face for an answer.

"Don't see how this is relevant," I said.

"Oh, of course not, just wondering," the doctor said hastily. "Looks like your vision won't be affected, but if you have any problems, give me a call."

I gathered my parka and wool hat. My palms sweated and I felt dizzy as I hurried towards the door. I stepped out into the ice-sharp, Alaskan air and the snow-glare blinded me. I put on my shades and took deep breaths. I began to walk home, crunching over the snow-crusted sidewalk as a syncopated rhythm drummed inside my head.

HIV SURVEY

THE FOLLOWING SURVEY is intended to provide critical information regarding transmission of the HIV virus. Please indicate the manner in which you believe you were exposed to HIV.

(check all that apply)

☒ blood transfusion
☒ mosquito
☒ evil dentist
☒ sex
☒ *promiscuous* sex
☒ sharing needles with drug-addicts
☒ having sex with drug-addicts
☒ doing drugs with sex-addicts
☒ a mosquito
☒ having sex with gay men
☒ sharing needles with gay men
☒ having sex with Haitians
☒ sharing needles with Haitians
☒ getting a blood transfusion from a Haitian
☒ a mosquito
☒ getting a blood transfusion from a gay man
☒ having sex with a blood transfusion recipient
☒ sharing needles with a blood transfusion recipient
☒ failing to accept Jesus Christ as your personal savior
☒ a mosquito

☒ having sex with someone who doesn't accept Jesus Christ as his personal savior

☒ sharing needles with someone who doesn't accept Jesus Christ as his personal savior

☒ a mosquito

☒ having promiscuous sex and sharing needles with a gay, Haitian, drug-using, sex-addicted, blood transfusion recipient who does not accept Jesus Christ as his personal savior.

☒ a mosquito

☒ all of the above

Rearranging the Furniture

In one recurring dream, Formosan termites eat through the soft wood of my house until the floors and walls weaken and collapse. I wake up to feel my heart racing. The next day a friend of mine looks up house images in her dream book and tells me that in dreams the house is one's body. I imagine my HIV medicines nesting inside my body, digging tunnels as they gnaw at the grain of my flesh, the veneer of my skin.

***

I had just turned thirty-seven when I first noticed a single, pronounced vein running down each of my arms. I realized that as my limbs grew thinner, the veins bulged into raised termite tunnels and lines criss-crossed down my legs like blue earthworm highways. On the backs of my calves tiny veins appeared like inky office doodles or badly drawn tattoos. I wondered if these veins were simply the hereditary gifts of my mother, or was the infamous AIDS wasting syndrome kicking in?

"Nice veins," the hospital phlebotomist says when I have blood drawn. She taps a vein on the inside of my arm, admires how it stands out, offers itself to the needle. I have noticed that if I become dehydrated, my veins stand out even more, as though the ebbing of an ocean of skin reveals the life below. It's hard for me to drink enough water because I get bored with the taste, so I drink lots of lemonade with mint to rehydrate, to help the tide wash back over the seaweed tangle of veins.

Meanwhile, my middle seems to thicken, but I am not sure if the changes are caused by genetics, age, HIV or the medicines; or perhaps it is just the perception of my body-conscious, American, female mentality.

***

I have been cleaning and decorating my 100-year-old New Orleans house in an attempt to control something in my life, as if straightening, cleaning, brightening can improve my body, cover the blue veins and bring color to my cheeks and eyes. I rearrange paintings and wall hangings as though this will counteract the effects of the drugs, make my limbs grow thicker and my torso thinner. I have lived with HIV for twelve years and have somehow managed to stay healthy—no pneumocystis pneumonia, Karposi sarcoma, thrush or the other frightening diseases that have plagued so many and that I fear. I have seen my t-cells rise over the years, and fortunately the medicines have suppressed my viral load to undetectable levels. I am grateful for these indications of good health, but then I glance down at my calves and try to read the blue hieroglyphics, possible side effects from years of taking nelfinavir, ritonavir, efavirenz, abacavir, didanosine.... .

***

I admire the cut flowers in the center of my dining room table. I like the way the red amaryllis complement the blue irises. I shift around the sunflowers and baby's breath until the cluster of color seems to radiate from the middle of the room. Then my eye catches the article on lipodystrophy in the copy of *Project Inform*, an AIDS journal of developments in medicine, that lies open on the table. I had been reading it earlier while I ate lunch.

The article discusses the side effects of various HIV drugs. This is when I begin to believe that my body is growing thinner as a side effect of my medicines. The protease inhibitor class of drugs can cause lipodystrophy or "truncating," where the fat redistributes, like a glacial migration, leaving the arms, legs, butt, and face thin, while the stomach and breasts grow larger. But I thought I only imagined these changes until recently.

***

"After a break-up, first thing, rearrange the furniture," my oldest sister Susan advised over the telephone after my boyfriend moved out.

I put on a *Talking Heads* CD—*More Songs about Buildings and Food*—and turned it up loud, percussion pounding to drown out my thoughts as I shoved and dragged beds and dressers around on blankets.

It seems like a feminine urge to shape and reshape our bodies and environment. I recently helped a friend haul a futon couch into her house, all the way to the back room that she uses as a home office. It was quite heavy and later we both had aching back muscles. When I returned the next evening to watch a video with her, she told me that she had single-handedly maneuvered that unwieldy futon back into the living room—she didn't like it in the office. I laughed at her for being so particular with her decorating scheme, even if it meant she had to haul furniture alone. She told me of a friend whose petite mother dragged a piano down a set of stairs by herself. I imagined the picnic-robbing ants in cartoons, a single one carrying a banana twenty times his size.

***

I angle my bed across a corner and then shove the chest of drawers in front of the tall window. I slide the dressing table by the other window and fill the empty drawers and shelves with all my stuff. I spread out my books and clothes as heart-rhythms thump in my head and chest. David Byrne and I chant: *"Here's-that-rhy-thm-again."*

I jump up and down to the song, roll my hips, and sing-shouting while my large black Labrador retrievers turn in circles and bark, bark, bark at me.

***

Every morning and evening, I take the pills out of the little pill containers that have days and times marked. I think of my late grandmother pushing her pills into piles with a frail finger. The easiest to take are the small blue or yellow capsules. The large, coffin-shaped, white chalky ones stick in my throat. The tiny pink ones shriek with bitterness, even if I wash them down with Coca-Cola. First thing in the morning, on an empty stomach, I chew four chalky, wafer-like double-quarter thick pills. I try to wash down the sticky residue with water as a river washes silt through a river bed. In my drowsy state, I barely notice the nasty-sweet taste.

The pills have names that sound like insect species and I imagine them climbing about in the overgrown garden in my front yard:

"The winged *Didanosine* thrives in tropical climates where it can be seen partying in Spanish Moss."

"With powerful mandibles the *Efavirenze* feeds primarily upon palmetto palm stalks and tastefully decorated old New Orleans homes."

"By injecting a nauseating venom, the *Ziagen* paralyzes its prey of beetles or streetcar passengers, then taunts its victims before sucking dry their life juices."

***

When I was a little girl, I listened to my older sisters and mom talk about their low-fat diets of fish and vegetables. My parents and sisters all seemed overweight at one time or another. But I can't distinguish the feelings from the reality. At nine years old, I felt left out so I would stick out my stomach and mimic, "I'm so fat."

"Don't joke," my sister Vikki said, "some day you may be." Perhaps I associated diets with womanhood.

I grew up feeling fat, though in retrospect, I suspect I was always average. But the small incidents cling to my imagination. I remember my Dad noticing my plump stomach hanging over my corduroy jeans and he suggested that I needed to lose a few pounds. A worried look showed in my mother's eyes one summer when she suggested I might want to go on a diet—"I don't want you to become obese," she said, and that word, *obese*, frightened me, as though I might grow into a grotesque, fat-jiggling, ground-shaking monstrosity. That night Mom invited me to go with her and Dad for ice cream and I remember resenting the mixed signals, but went anyway and ordered a Swenson's pink peppermint cone rolled in chocolate jimmies. My parents went out for ice cream almost every night in those days.

When I was twelve years old, my sister Susan said that if I lost ten pounds she would buy me a bikini, an idea that delighted me. I think I only lost seven, but she took me shopping at J.C. Penny's anyway, and I wore that emerald green bikini for two summers before I could no longer deny that my body had developed out of it, no matter how tightly I tied the top. But most of my adult life I struggled with my cravings for rich foods like ice cream and buttery rolls, which inevitably brought about thick thighs and a flabby stomach.

When my long-term boyfriend moved out, he left bare spaces on my book shelves, in closets and drawers, the rooms of my house and in the corners of my days. The break-up was a familiar one: after five and a half years together, I wanted something more permanent, and he didn't. I asked him if fear of HIV kept him from staying. He said no, he just wasn't ready to make a commitment. I asked him to move out, which he did quickly and efficiently.

About a month later, I looked into the bathroom mirror one morning and noticed the usual morning wrinkles that crease the left side of my face, the side on which I sleep. Then I saw dark patches on my cheeks as if an impressionist painter had smudged a solid blue-gray patch beneath each of my cheek bones. I tried to wash with soap and water, but the dark areas remained. I thought the room too dark, so I turned on the overhead light, then the lights that encircle my bathroom mirror, and I leaned closer, but the dark shadows still clung to the chiseled landscape of my face. I didn't understand. I knew I had been eating less in my new loneliness, and the swampy summer heat robbed my appetite. I had not yet turned on my air-conditioner, because the summer electric bills are very high in these drafty old southern homes. I found my own drawn face frightening. This sudden thinning was surely unnatural. Concern over weight loss was one I had never experienced in my life. After all, as a young American female, I had learned the mantra early on: *Thinner is better, thinner is better, thinner is better.* Was it time to learn to wear the makeup I'd shunned all of my life in a desperation to hide my real, hollow-cheeked face? My mind flashed to the faces of evening news AIDS victims with corpse-stares. Had my face become so emaciated, my head a skull with wild Halloween hair? My own mortality stared back at me through a sunken-eyed skull-face. Eventually I sat down at the table and began a shopping list of fatty foods to buy and a list of house chores.

***

Take out the dust mop and sweep the soft dark clumps of dog hair into a pile. (There is hair enough to stuff a dozen pillows.) Dust the shelves, file bills, maps, travel brochures. Put photos in photo albums, put away letters, cut and tape recipes onto file cards.

***

I have always wanted to be one of those women who can eat anything she wants without gaining weight. When I first noticed myself thinning, my stomach sickened with alarm, but then I began the hedonistic eating orgy of which I have always dreamed. I went out to Mexican restaurants to eat cheesy enchiladas, chalupas, flautas, burritos and chimichangas, and sopapillas dripping with honey. I ordered regular cokes, spooned honey into my tea, and munched popcorn with butter at the movies. I stocked my refrigerator with sour cream and cheeses. I stuffed Dove dark chocolate ice cream bars in the freezer and munched greasy Zapp's potato chips with my sandwiches. I didn't gain weight and have continued to indulge. I devour delicious food with the same pleasure I take drinking in vivid colors of cut flowers and the bright shades of paintings in my house, I take it all in.

It seems that I have two contradictory inclinations. On one hand, I try to keep control of the interior of my house, as I try to control the disease and the appearance of my body. And yet living in doubt of my future, I want to indulge myself, to live my life as fully as possible for I crave delicious foods, music, flowers, art and sex.

***

I had a fine date with a handsome man a few weeks ago, and as he and I sat on my couch, becoming romantic, I felt energized. He massaged my feet and admired my cobalt-blue painted toe nails. He ran his piano-player long fingers over my bare, tan summer-legs, complimenting my calves. I felt a glow as he stroked my calves, felt as though the beauty of

64

my home flowed into my body that night. I hadn't yet told him that I was HIV positive—he only knew that he was wooing me, could have no idea that he was soothing a particular part of my body that I had begun to feel anxiety over. He didn't seem to notice the blue veins. This sexy moment returned to me the feeling of being vibrant, human, normal.

***

My old bras have become too snug, the next size larger a neat fit. Perhaps if I were a skinny, small-breasted woman I would be grateful to fill out my figure. But I already feel self-conscious. As I walk down the street, sometimes I believe I notice men staring at my chest and I feel like I am a sex freak, a pair of breasts walking around on spindly legs.

A couple of years ago when I was vacationing in Charlotteville, Tobago, a native woman told me people in town had been discussing me, the American, noting how unusual it was that I was so small, with large breasts. I imagined people laughing over glasses of rum in steamy bars, gossipy women chopping fish and plantains at kitchen tables, sweaty talkative fishermen in the market, all talking about the body that I thought was personal, mine. At times I feel as if I am in one of those dreams where I am nude, parading proudly in a florescent-lit shopping mall or hiding from co-workers behind office furniture.

***

I primp and stare, tracing the deep creases in my face. I wonder if my worry shows. I suppose it is a sign of progress when I feel more concerned about the effects the drugs have on my appearance than the effects of the disease—when I fret over my looks, instead of merely trying to cling to my health, my life. Perhaps this vanity, brushing my hair in front of the mirror, painting my toe nails bright colors, flaunting slender white sandals and a glittering silver anklet, is a part of being alive. Or do I fixate on these superficial concerns to avoid thinking too deeply about the virus that courses through my veins, and swarms throughout my body?

In casual conversation at work one day, I told Sandra, our department secretary, that I felt good having written a poem. I admitted I had felt depressed the day before.

"Why were you depressed, Trecie?" she asked. I realized I had said too much and she knew something was wrong. I suspected she had noticed my worried look and thinning body. I felt frightened at that moment, to be so vulnerable, so visible.

"I've just been tired," I told her. "You can tell?"

"You wear it," she said. "You wear it."

I felt embarrassed, and wondered if she might think I wear my emotions on purpose.

I wished to hide at that moment. But I have never been able to hide my feelings. I laugh loudly during Steve Martin movies, smile open-mouthed during a spirited brass band parade, and grin into my partner's face when I Zydeco dance—but I cry easily when I feel sad. I was afraid I would break into tears, and felt the urge to reassure her there was no need to worry.

"Tell me what's wrong, please," she said as her kind brown eyes looked into mine.

"I think it's just the heat." I shifted in my chair. "I finally turned on my air last week, shouldn't have waited so long."

"Well," she said as I stood to leave, "people are very concerned about you."

With the word "people," I imagined small meetings where friends talked about my body changes and once again I felt that nude-in-public-dream feeling.

As friends and colleagues continued to confront me one by one, I felt turned inside out like a mango peel, my emotions exposed and pulpy. I didn't know who to talk to or what to say. If I had discussed the ex-boyfriend, I would have burst into tears like a lovesick teenager, right there in the office. If I had mentioned that I have HIV, I was afraid these concerned friends would have panicked. And I wondered if my department chair or colleagues would question my ability to do my job.

They might fear I was contagious and avoid sharing office space, pens, or a dessert over lunch. What might my colleagues imagine as the cause of my subdued behavior and weight loss? Clinical depression? Breast cancer? Ovarian cancer? I felt a need to protect not only myself, but to protect friends from worry. I didn't want to be thought of as a person who burdens others with my problems or craves sympathy.

But the worries of others increased my own, and at the time I didn't know why I was thinning. My change in appearance alarmed me, during a summer when I was scoping out possible new romances at clubs and parties, trying to fill the empty shelves in my love life.

***

Hang the beaded voodoo flags; polish the leather-covered coffee table; put the green table cloth and straw place mats on the table; dust ceiling fan blades, grandma's ship-wheel clock, and the stained glass lamp; put marigolds in the cranberry glass, a rose in the glass bud vase; straighten pictures: Native American abstracts with bright cubist faces, huge 6 x 4 primitive paintings with blue people, fire-eyed dogs, burning buildings. Burn "desert rain" incense, wash the dog-nose smudges off the windows.

***

Reverend Harris, my next door neighbor, has Alzheimer's disease and a nurse takes care of him every day. His wife, Mrs. Harris, is frail and stays inside the house most of the time. The nurse and Mr. Harris sit on the front porch together, but she gets restless, goes into the yard to push the lawn mower and clip the edges of the lawn. One day she cut the new shoots of my rose bush that grew through the chain-link fence into the Harris' yard. I glared at her, told her that if Mrs. Harris didn't want the roses growing on her side of the fence, I would gladly put up a partition. But Mrs. Harris had told *me* she didn't mind. I had been nourishing the bush, giving it fertilizer and mulching around the roots. Whenever I cut the crimson buds to bring into the house I carefully clipped down to the junction, as my mother had instructed me, so that the bush would produce new growth. In my fury over the snipped shoots, I considered putting up a trellis, or an ugly bamboo fence between us. Maybe a gray cinder block wall.

"So sorry," the nurse said, but she didn't look sorry. She kept tugging at untidy weeds by the front fence. I noticed she had even dug up the begonias and day lilies that had lined the Harris's house. As Mr. Harris sat strapped in his wheel chair arguing with visions of deceased relatives, she stabbed a pointed shovel into the garden, daring anything green ever to grow in that soil again.

Nurse Kill-It-All squatted low to pull, clip and shovel, as she began to tell me about her sick sister with liver cancer, and a nephew with sickle-cell anemia. She said working in the yard gave her mind ease. Loose flesh jiggled beneath her busy arms as she tugged and trimmed and clipped, mourning hopeless situations that rooted in her mind. Meanwhile, she was snipping the yard into a sharp-edged square, neat as a new place mat.

She tried to cut back wild growth, to limit the green life, as I was trying to nourish and promote new growth. However, tropical plants flourish out of control in my yard. Greenery grows and tangles as thickly as an Amazon jungle. It might not be surprising to see an anaconda uncoil from beneath the thicket of wild petunias, or to witness a jaguar peering down from the roof through the dark rubber tree branches. An anarchy of white ginger blooms springs upward like a fragrant geyser. In the night, the sweet scents of the ginger, the night-blooming jasmine and the Angel's Trumpet compete and overwhelm the air. If I didn't cut the grass soon, I might need a machete to hack my way from my doorstep, through the small front yard and to my truck each morning.

I decided against the cinder-block wall and Nurse-Machete never clipped at the shoots of my rose bush again.

***

In another dream, a tremendous thunderstorm pours water into my house through the holes in the roof. I look for the phone number of the roofing company that had just installed the new roof, but can't find it. A worker had been walking on the roof and left piles of slate, the job unfinished. I feel angry and helpless in this dream.

***

As a teenager, I attended an expensive, private high school with tall, slender, *Vogue*-beautiful girls. I thought of myself as plain and unfeminine. By the time we were seniors, several of my friends had fought bouts of anorexia. I remember one girl as stocky and athletic, another full-faced and beautiful. Then one by one, each began dieting, until their energy and beauty had drained away, leaving terribly thin, frail girls. I felt disturbed and worried about them. As for me, on one hand I felt rebellious against the pressure to be thin. And yet I too was haunted by the tall, waif-like ideal of beauty. This ideal crept into our minds as we flipped through shiny glamour magazine ads, overheard the comments of our peers and parents, and watched the popular, high-cheek-boned beauties who sauntered about during morning assembly.

As I look at myself in a full-length mirror, my thick, self-image competes with my concern over my skinny butt and legs. I can't remember how I used to really look, or see how I look now. I see image upon image like a pile of transparencies, based on what I hear from my friends and family, and what I *think* I see in the mirror, what I *think* I remember I looked like years ago. My stomach has always protruded, like my mother's—is it more distended now? My childhood friend Trinica says I've always had skinny arms and legs, though I know the bulging veins are new. She says I just look like I workout, and this thought comforts me. My mother has "chicken legs" with blue veins. I can't distinguish with any certainty the results of aging, drug side effects, my natural body type, depression over a lost love, or my fickle memory and imagination.

***

I cover my legs with citronella bug repellant before I go outside to weed the garden, trim night-blooming jasmine, wash the dogs and comb their fur so they will shine. I transplant coral-blossom Angel's Trumpet, hang baskets of yellow walking iris, baskets of fuscia desert rose, baskets of crimson begonias. The small, tiger-mosquitoes buzz hungrily around my ankles.

***

In the summer that the boyfriend moved out, the summer of a sweaty house, rearranged furniture, empty shelves and fresh hollows in my face, I went to a small family reunion at my parents' house in Santa Fe, New Mexico. I was nervous about the journey, wishing I could disguise the diminutive self I had become and hide from my parents and two sisters. They, of course, knew of my having HIV for all these years, but I always felt the impulse to protect them. I did not mention to my family a cold that lingered too long; I did not mention fears of ending up in the hospital. Only with hesitation would my mother ask about my health, and only reluctantly would I offer information. I tried to tell her mostly of positive signs, such as rising T-cells or good health, despite my working with sickly colleagues during flu season.

When I arrived in Albuquerque for the reunion, I walked past the crowd of turquoise-jeweled strangers to the baggage claim carousel. My bag was one of the last ones to come up the chute, and just as I hauled the strap over my shoulder my mom appeared. She approached with a smile, but it looked to me like her eyes were studying my face and body. She hugged me tight and then began complaining that my father made them late because he had to stop at the post office to mail some packages, that Dad said it wouldn't take very long, but it did. He was waiting in the red Nissan Pathfinder, parked in the five minute zone. Their Malamute mix, Stormy, looked out the back with dark ringed eyes. Dad stepped out and hugged me, his beard scratchy against my face. His pool-green eyes looked tired, surrounded by a Sahara of wrinkles. Dad took my bag and put it in the back with Stormy. The one-and-a-half hour long drive to Santa Fe was quiet, with sparse, cautious conversation.

"How was your flight? Uneventful, I hope," my father said.

"Fine," I said, as Stormy drooled on my shoulder.

"Those jeans got pretty loose on you," my mother said, glancing back at me.

"Lost some weight," I said.

"Wish *I* had that problem," Dad said as he whipped into the left lane and sped towards Santa Fe. My father doesn't ask about my health often, nor mention any body changes that he may notice. He settles into a serene cloud of silence, broken by occasional questions or smart-ass comments.

As we talked I could hear strands of concern in my mother's voice, even as she chatted about the wild flowers that had bloomed in her yard. My mother is comforted by a flurry of chatter. Mom described virtually every single gray jay, junco, bluebird, yellow warbler, gold finch, black-capped chickadee, and red-breasted grosbeak that had landed on her bird feeder in the past month as my father swung in and out of lanes with his death-defying Indianapolis 500 driving style. Her bird monologue was punctuated by an occasional gasp, which my father pretended not to hear.

Since this weight loss was uncharacteristic for me, I was glad for any distraction.

We arrived at the house to the hugs, smiles and wise-ass cutting up that my family revels in. But my sister Susan changed the tone with, "You've lost a lot of weight."

My aunt looked me over, but she didn't appear concerned—she didn't know I had HIV.

I began to tell Sue about the heat and humidity, but she wasn't listening, she never does. Her eyes filled with panic as she said again, "You lost a lot of weight, Trece'."

I tried to use a casual tone to tell her about the boyfriend-depression, but I knew she was thinking about AIDS.

Susan led me into the back bedroom and shut the door.

"It's the drugs that do this, Sue," I said, "that make me lose weight, my doctor doesn't know what to do about it."

"You know, working out with weights can help with wasting... ," she interrupted.

I became angry that she dared use that word "wasting"—a word I associate with AIDS, hospitals, dying. I was annoyed that she didn't hear my explanation and we retreated into a familiar, stubborn, sisterly standoff, this time born of concern, frustration, and love.

We seemed so far from the day she had rewarded me with that bright green bikini. "Thin" used to mean healthy, beautiful and successful in my family, but now it suggested "AIDS Victim."

***

"Look at this," I show my doctor the veins in my legs.

He notices the blue lines on my calves, as well as the creases in my face. We spend little time discussing my T-cell count, which has risen from 139 to 278 in the past year, and viral load remains undetectable. I beg for solutions to these body changes.

My doctor nods, but doesn't have an answer. Researchers aren't sure of the reasons for the lipodystrophy and there is controversy over exactly which drug combinations cause this wasting effect. He tells me about some studies that will begin in the coming months and then hesitantly suggests I try eating more fats. I think it's difficult for him to give this kind of advice, as he is health-oriented. I imagine him jogging several times a week and eating mostly lean meats and steamed vegetables.

"I do eat fat," I say, and then run through the list of Mexican foods I have been devouring.

He smiles.

I still feel frustrated by my appearance and I don't tell him about my growing urge to attract handsome men into my life. It is not always food that I crave.

***

Glue arm back on the kachina doll, polish cypress fireplace mantles (1/3 linseed oil, 1/3 turpentine, 1/3 vinegar), wipe down base boards, wash, dry and fold clothes, iron skirts, run the dishwasher and put away plates, scrub soap scum off the royal blue bath tiles.

***

I planted seedlings at the start of the summer, and now I have three sunflower plants, only one of which is blooming. The flower has a large black disk center and blazing yellow petals. The marigolds are just about to open, and a hanging basket overflows with hot pink portulaca. I have piled cedar chips in the front garden to keep the soil moist. I brought home a full bouquet from the store—there are not yet enough blooms in the garden to cut and I fuss over getting the right balance of reds, yellows and blues in the vase.

My life feels like borrowed time and I crave a heightened sense of experience. I want to devour colors, flavors, music, textures, scents, elements that make me feel more human.

***

When I was in 8th grade, I drew a collection of pen and ink drawings, which I showed my art teacher, Mr. Rudari. He complimented the line quality. One of the drawings was of an electrical outlet with vines and feathers growing out of the sockets. Mr. Rudari said he thought the drawing represented my sexuality coming forth. He explained that an outlet represented female anatomy and said the plants represented my blossoming sensuality. At sixteen, I blushed and discounted his explanation; it was just a cool drawing to me. But now, I feel that I am that outlet with electricity and greenery springing forth out of my life. I believe this sensitivity and sexuality makes me feel most alive. And I hope to hold onto the power that flows like the blood in my veins, despite surging threats of illness.

With the improvement of my health, my demands for quality-of-life grow like the cries of a spoiled child: I want a smooth face, and bigger legs and arms. I resent the blue squiggle veins. I suppose I am trying to postpone mortality and hold onto my youth and life long enough to embrace a future.

I let the yard bloom into a mass of tangled growth in the summer rains. I crave the flavors of rich foods, and wish to fill my home with vivid, colorful flowers. A Samba beat blasts from my stereo speakers and the scent of night blooming jasmine oozes in through the doors and windows. The sounds drive me to dance around my kitchen and sing as I stir a pot of curried lamb. I want to smell spices and incense, feel the touch of rose petals, or a man's hands massaging the bottom of my foot. I think this greed is a natural tendency for me. When I think of the HIV crouching inside my body, my drive for life intensifies until I am immersed in the days of heat and colors.

Conversation with a Heroin Addict

Walter handed me a Granny Smith apple and a tin of Moroccan sardines in pepper oil—courting gifts. 8:00 a.m. I took them and set them on the table.

Walter and I sat on my yellow and rose flowered couch, laughing. He had come by to pick up his electric saw, and without invitation he plopped down on my couch. I sat as far from him as possible. Faded red socks, black tennis shoes, filthy white shorts. Grey-rot teeth. Cigarette butt dead on the table. His thick eyebrows furrowed in concentration as he tried to formulate a question.

"I wanted to ask you the other night about HIV and sex. I'd been thinking about you." Walter was a carpenter and did some work for me replacing the rotten weather boards along the side of my house. But he seemed to want to know me better and lingered after his work was done. I had told him that I had HIV, thinking I could conveniently deter him. But he lingered all the same.

I explained only about the pills I took.

"But how do you know you have it?" He reached for my knee.

I recoiled.

"Have you been retested?" he asked.

I told him that I had been tested twice. I added that luckily, my viral load remained undetectable but over the years my t-cells fell from a normal 800 to around 250. I described the Interleuken II study that interested me, a treatment that might raise a person's t-cells. But I didn't want to take part in the study; it would require injections. I hate needles.

"You can't give yourself a little shot?" he asked.

I grimaced.

"It's easy," he said. "I'm a heroin addict, you know, my veins have all collapsed. I haven't shot up in years, but it's easy!" He took my hand, turned my palm up. "Piece a cake." He traced the veins on the underside of my forearm. "You couldn't do that?"

"Can't stand pain!" I pulled my hand out of his. "You gotta do it twice a day for five days."

"You ain't no baby. I'd do it for you," he said.

I considered the intimacy, almost sexual, of letting a friend insert a needle beneath your skin. I know nothing about the culture of addicts, but I assume it would involve pain and would require trust. Letting a friend slide a needle into my vein would differ from my visits to the medical clinic. There, I hold out my arm for a phlebotomist to wrap the rubber strap around my upper arm; the needle enters the vein and blood rises into the syringe. Although she is not my personal friend, I trust her to hit the vein the first time, quickly, with compassion.

"There's probably guys all over the neighborhood who could help me out," I said.

"Sure," Walter laughed. "Just go down to Jackson Ave., say, 'Hey buddy, I give you five bucks a pop.'" Jackson Avenue was a rough area where I had seen men and women sitting on sidewalks, backs up against the wall of an abandoned building, staring with vacant eyes.

I imagined telling my doctor that I wanted to join the Interleuken II study. "I have this friend who would be happy to assist me with the shots. He's a junkie, well, not anymore, an ex-junkie, really, hasn't shot up since the 70s, but I bet he'd still be pretty good at it. I suspect it's like riding a bicycle, once you learn…" I would promise that we would not share needles. I imagined the office, clean white surfaces and my doctor's young, attentive, sincere face. He would try not to look shocked so as not to alienate the patient.

"Hang tough," Walter plugged a cigarette out on my floor and stood up to leave. "Let me kiss your AIDS-tinged cheek," he said, but I pulled back just in time. He raised one eyebrow, then walked out the door.

Dating Exam

I WANTED A BOYFRIEND, and needed contractors to make repairs on my house. The contractors seemed to be applying for the job of boyfriend. When a painter or carpenter finished a job for me, he looked around and offered to hang a picture, install dimmer switches or replace a rotted weather board—anything to linger a little longer. In order to kill two birds with one stone, I developed the following exam to help me evaluate men who might be good boyfriends and could also help me make repairs to my house.

Documentation Required:
drug test
certification of sanity
building permit
driving record
credit report
bank statement
green card (as needed)
brake tag
rabies tag

Multi-task Skills Test: **Perform any five of the Following Tasks in a 24 hour period:**
Fix a running toilet
Put on a condom
Write a movie scene in which a bottle of wine is not drunk (nor is the person.)

Install, caulk and paint a weatherboard
Watch a foreign film
Refill an ice cube tray
Fix a leaky roof
Call NO/AIDs Task Force hot line and ask a question about HIV
Drive a standard shift car
Speak to a woman without leering or lapsing into a condescending tone
Shake hands with a gay man
Read a book or newspaper
Turn off a television
Wipe pee off the rim of the toilet
Lay tile
Listen without interrupting
Replace a window pane

Dating Test: **With which of the following statements do you agree?**

Condoms, yeah! Mix and match, colors and flavors!
Prayer in school should be mandatory.
Algebra classes in church should be mandatory
Condoms make my wee wee shrivel up.
Women who have had more than an 8th grade education make my wee
       wee shrivel up.
Sometimes I hear voices.
I would rather eat a limp, cold tofu burger than a T-bone steak.
Communication is for wusses.
I can smash a beer can against my forehead.
I's smashed jillion's o' dem cans 'gainst my head.
Meeting a woman with HIV would be fine.
The way things have been going lately, getting HIV or swallowing a bottle
       of sleeping pills, it's all the same to me.
Nixon made some good points, just had a bad rap.

Circle any of the following that you concern you:

Power lines, phone lines, movie lines, copper pans, milk, meat, plants, fungus, airplanes, cars, apocalypse, germs, caffeine, hormone induced meat, hot house tomatoes, The Rolling Stones, Total Ozone Depletion, the second coming, rap music, foreign languages or accents, religions other than your own, other skin/eye/hair color, non-organic veggies, non-macrobiotic foods, small spaces, cracks in the sidewalk, whistling in the wheel house, nematodes, radiated fruits and vegetables, immunizations, modern medicine, herbal medicine, UFO-abduction.

Other: _____

Demonstrate competence using the following tools:

Circular saw
hand saw
hammer
drill
street map
paint brush
condom

Extra Credit (5 points each):

Shore up a house.
Honor a birthday other than your own.
Tell a joke that doesn't include the word "pussy."

For Office Use Only

criminal record
racist
sexist
armed
xenophobic
alcoholic
abuser

sex addict
celibate
drug addict
polygamous
suicidal
paranoid
jail bait
homophobic
phobic
other

owns car that runs
attracted
attractive
literate
fluent in at least one language
monogamous
relationship oriented
witty
condom literacy

Test Scores

HIV knowledge
technical HIV skills
imaginative skills
social skills
technical maintenance skills

Holding the Wheel

On my 16th birthday, my father drove me to the Texas Department of Public Safety to take the driving exam. It was a Saturday, and Dad brought me to the office in Richardson, Texas, about 45 minutes from where we lived. Only the Richardson office stayed open on Saturday. We went in Dad's red MGB, which had black leather seats that were so deep, I had to sit on a telephone book to see over the dashboard.

At the Department of Motor Vehicles, I got in the car with the evaluator, who grasped a clipboard and pencil, and I started the car. When I pressed the gas and let up on the clutch, the car lurched forward and the engine died. The evaluator told me I had left the parking brake on. I restarted, pulled up hard on the brake lever between the seats, pushed the release with my thumb, then lowered the lever. The rest of the test went better, and I passed, barely. Dad let me drive the car, on that bright sunny city day, with the top down; and the car engine rumbled powerfully as I raced over the smooth streets of Dallas. To me, driving meant freedom. A strong wind tangled my wavy mass of hair, and heat radiated up from the cement.

One Saturday that summer, I stood with my dad in the K-Mart parking lot watching his friends maneuver their sports cars around a course marked by orange cones. Dad urged me to try to drive the auto cross that was organized by the Dallas Sports Car Club. The idea was to drive the maze-like route as quickly as possible without knocking over any orange cones. I found the route confusing and I feared that I would lose my way. I rode in the passenger seat while Dad drove through it once. Orange cones seemed to pop up like bright flashing warnings in a video game as Dad steered the car hard to the right, hard left, weaving, swerving until we finished and I felt even more disoriented. I said I didn't want to drive the course. "That's okay," Dad said, and we went home.

To my father, driving meant responsibility. He believed that people didn't need to learn to drive more slowly, they needed to learn to drive better. He joked that most driver exams in the U.S. amounted to the examiner holding up a mirror to the applicant's face and if the mirror fogged, the driver passed the test and was awarded a license. Dad admired the more rigorous driving tests of France and Britain. But in many European cities, people can rely on efficient public transportation systems, networks of undergrounds, tubes, double decker buses and cross-country, high-speed rail systems. Although I liked to drive, I also envied those with other options, who could get by without a car and sidestep the responsibility. Dad felt people needed to know how to swerve out of the way of reckless drivers without running into someone else. He had read about driving schools in California where they strap a helmet to your head, put you into a race car with good roll bars, buckle your seat belt and they direct you to slide around over wet or icy pavement. You learn how to steer your car out of a spin and find out how hard you can turn before the car rolls. But when you complete training, you can really handle a car. Dad said that if he could afford it, he would like to send me to this kind of school.

I have developed an overly-strong sense of responsibility that comes to play when I think about how I acquired HIV. I am hyper-aware of the factors that are within my control. I tend to disregard factors beyond my control and forget about my human fallibility, the margin of error.

***

A group of twenty-five Central African Republic Peace Corps Volunteers watched the demonstration as Abigail unrolled a yellow condom over the end of a broomstick. "This is for those of you interested in sampling the 'local talent,'" she said. Some of us giggled, I don't remember if I did or not. I was young, healthy, twenty-three years old. I already knew how to use condoms. But I was used to men who shunned them. I remembered an ex-boyfriend who had said that using a condom was like "coming into a plastic bag." I went on the pill and rarely used condoms. I was warned that HIV existed in the Central African region. The man who gave it to me didn't know he had it. It doesn't matter anymore, but a sense of responsibility slips back into my consciousness.

***

When I heard that Vincent had died of AIDS, a shiver climbed my spine. It was December and I was home from graduate school for the holidays. Mary Ellen, a Peace Corps administrator, told me about it as she tried to contact another volunteer who had dated him. If she knew that I had been involved with him, she did not say so.

"By the way, how are you feeling?" she asked. She knew I had HIV from when I was diagnosed.

"Fine," I said. "I read that there are people who never develop symptoms. I figure, maybe I could be one of those people."

"Patrice," Mary Ellen said. "Oh Patrice …"

I hung up the phone.

I had been involved with Vincent only briefly, during the Peace Corps training in Bambari, Central African Republic. I remember Vincent's tall, tautly muscled frame, high cheek bones and flirtatious eyes. He was one of the French and Sango language teachers. He also was a tailor and sometimes sewed clothes for a number of Peace Corps volunteers. I saw him in my mind as he measured yards of deep purple fabric; he ran soft folds between his thumb and forefinger for a *boubou* he was making me. I had picked out a light cotton with a bright green floral and parrot pattern over the midnight purple. I liked the way the finished *boubou* draped over my arms and legs like a breezy waterfall.

I had been diagnosed with HIV seven months before this phone call, through a series of routine blood tests. I did not know from whom I got it. There were a couple of men I had dated during my Peace Corps stay. But when I was first diagnosed, I was focused on myself as I mourned my condition and my parents tried to comfort me, though they mourned too. It was strange to have a face to associate with HIV. Panic flashed inside of me and I wondered when my body would begin to die. I didn't tell anyone about Vincent or what Mary Ellen had said.

I lost my appetite. I couldn't eat the plates of yellow squash and roast beef Mom served, and I couldn't tell her why. I wanted to talk to someone about my fears and what I had learned about Vincent. But to tell my parents or friends would contribute to their own anxieties, and this would increase my own.

***

I had one of my first car accidents while driving my Dad's MG. I was lucky to be allowed to drive my parents' speedy foreign cars. I was still sixteen years old and I drove in the center lane headed for the North Dallas Toll Road to go home. My school friend and neighbor Lydia was with me.

A brown Buick worked its way across two lanes of frantic 4:00 p.m. traffic to merge onto the toll road but the driver didn't see the little red MG and she slammed sideways into us. Both cars came to a stop and traffic stalled all around us.

"It's–not–your–fault," Lydia said calmly, with certainty. But I knew this argument wouldn't work in my household. If I failed to anticipate the car about to change lanes, honk loudly and zip out of the way, it was my fault. I had seen each of my alert, quick-reflexed parents avoid collisions. That evening, my annoyed parents took away my driving rights for a couple months. They felt they had endured enough car damage and insurance rate hikes.

Lessons of responsibility have become a part of my fabric.

Maggots of guilt eat away inside me.

***

The first time I saw a person dying was in the Central African Republic when a man named Engime, a fellow professor of geography in Bangassou, became ill. When I visited him in the hospital, I didn't recognize the skeleton-thin man lying on the bed with his limbs angled awkwardly. He trembled, struggling to move an arm or foot. The dry season had set in and the heat and dust baked the room. His head curved like a brown eggshell with veins about to crack open. I could almost see the pain in his temples racing to his skull and jaw. His skin hung loosely about his bones, and he riveted his hands to his head as if trying to grip the pain. He rocked back and forth to the throbbing and his toes grasped the wrinkles in his unmade bed. As the sheets slid off, one of his colleagues tucked them back around the edges of the foam mattress. I became dizzy. In the long room full of ailing people, I leaned against the molting, salmon-colored wall. Flakes of dead paint fell against the back of my neck. Six beds lined the walls and two stood in the middle of the room. I could smell the smoke of cooking fires outside as families prepared daily meals for loved ones in the hospital. His colleague said he would go to the country to find traditional medicine. I nodded though I doubted he could be saved.

Engime died a week later and I went to the funeral with another Peace Corps volunteer. I remember seeing the body laid out on a bed, low to the ground, and his family gathered around him, moaning softly. Even in the dim light, his skull looked polished. His cold, brass-toned forehead reflected the candlelight, and the small flames burned like half moons on either side of his face. A sheet covered the rest of his body and bunched up under his arms like bleached cow hide. In the weeks that followed his death, some professors guessed that he died of tuberculosis. A fellow Peace Corps Volunteer speculated AIDS.

Years later, I see in my mind the long-bodied corpse, and I see Engime's face, then Vincent's face, then Engime, then Vincent. Vincent had died of AIDS, and so would I, I thought. I wondered if my face would grow thin and corpse-like. I felt like hitting the "escape" key on the computer keyboard to exit this life-and-death, glad-and-depressed program. But the screen had frozen up. The curser wouldn't move and I cursed my situation, I cursed myself.

***

As I sat on my bedroom rug, I thought of Vincent and tried to reassure myself that I would be fine. In those days, I searched for hope as I perused news articles about people who had beaten the odds and remained asymptomatic for years. I remember a story about frozen blood samples from years ago, some of which contained the AIDS virus, and many of the infected individuals were still living, ten or fifteen years later.

***

Some people deny responsibility like those who regularly have conflicts with co-workers and never recognize a pattern. Such a person does not see his own contribution to the argument—it is always the other person's fault. At the other extreme are people who feel at fault for everything and everyone, such as a mother may feel for the behavior of her teenage children, or a friend's unhappiness. This person always wonders, "Maybe there was something more I could have done to help." I lean towards the latter category. I can't seem to let go of the recognition that I could have used a condom and did not. I could have refused to have unsafe sex, could have sacrificed convenience. In my mind, I am always driving the car. I cannot control the other drivers, the weather, driving conditions or the traffic lights. But my hands hold the steering wheel. However it comforts me to see the guilt-responsibility balance in different ways. It helps me to take a look at the many factors at play that might affect my marred driving record. But my humanly-flawed, living guilt corrodes my stomach like battery acid.

***

In Central Africa, all around me lived people who were ill with preventable or curable conditions such as malnutrition, malaria or schistosomiasis, but they lacked access to treatment. There was Ndoli, the skinny, 13-year old boy who had knobby, polio-weakened legs. Ndoli's straw hat tilted at an angle above a mischievous smile. He laughed and hobbled deftly on one crutch in a neighborhood game of soccer, slicing at the ball with the crutch. Next door lived my leprosy-ridden neighbor. When I returned home after a long journey, the old woman called me to her and held my hands between her cool hard hands, smooth stumps for fingers. She cradled my face between pebbled palms. Some evenings I saw her wearing cone-shaped cups the size of shot glasses suctioned to her back, chest and arms to suck out the evil spirits. Children walked to school with hungry, distended bellies. Occasionally I might notice a woman walking back from her field, short wooden hoe over her shoulder, a bucket of cassava on her head and an apple-sized goiter lump at her throat from lack of iodine. People suffered from *curable* diseases; I was not thinking about AIDS.

***

"Things just happen," said my friend Randi twenty years later. "You can't control *everything*." Randi thought my father's driving lessons harsh, especially for a child. "Sometimes another car will hit you and there is nothing you can do," she says.

Randi said the same of HIV. She reminds me that lots of people have unprotected sex. Some who use protection slip up from time to time. Not all partners have HIV and not all partners who do, pass it on. Anyone can get HIV. No one is perfect, and I was unlucky, she reminds me.

When I lived in the Central African Republic, I recall that people held a stronger sense of fate. If it rained, no one showed up for a coffee rondevous, or even a business appointment. Most of the communities had no telephones with which to keep in touch so if you missed appointments, it was understood. Many people felt that whatever happened was God's will. In our hyper-communicative North American society, our lives fill with the beeps, rings and buzzes of home phones, car phones, cell phones, electronic pagers, answering machines, blackberries, phone mails, e-mail and faxes. There's almost no excuse not to call if you are running late or can't make a meeting. At times these modes of communication overwhelm me, leave little excuse to be out of touch, free for a spontaneous moment. I think these conveniences create an illusion of total control and it becomes difficult to accept the multitude of factors that complicate a situation. I can understand how unrealistic the expectation of complete control in life, yet I still carry this guilt in my gut. When I feel my life reeling out of control, I hear my dad's instructions to watch out for cars that could sideswipe me. Then I hear Lydia proclaim, "It's—not—your—fault." I want to accept my errors and lack of control. But deep trenches or regret resonate and logic falls at the foothills of my emotion. I wish I knew how to dissolve this unsettling song that vibrates in my gut.

DATING AND MARRIAGE

THE NEVILLE BROTHERS

I HAD BECOME FASCINATED with the Neville Brothers' new album, *Yellow Moon,* which I played on my little boom box every night when I got home from grad school classes in Alaska. I turned the volume up loud and danced around the living room, grooving with Kufaru Mouton's heavy conga drum beats on "My Blood," digging Charles Neville's haunting saxophone rifts.

I was about to graduate that year and it was time for me to find work. I wondered what I would do if I didn't get a job after I graduated? I wondered, *What if I sent out thirty or fifty applications, as my professors expected of me, and got nothing?*

This was my secret desire.

I could see it, me in a pickup truck, everything I owned in the back and I would just drive and drive until the land flattened out, then filled with water; I would drive until I found myself flying over steaming, stenching swamps, until I saw curtains of morning fog.

Louisiana had pulled me towards her for years, from the time I first volunteered as a DJ on Blue Monday in a university basement, on the frozen Fairbanks campus.

"This is Blue Monday on KUAC-FM," I said into the microphone, but when I went back into the record stacks, my fingers kept skipping over Charlie Musslewhite and dug into James Booker, Professor Long Hair, Dr. John, Marcia Ball, Clifton Chenier, Johnny Adams and then the Nevilles started digging into me, Aaron's sweet high voice kept calling, Mean Willie Green drove those drums like wind drives a thunderstorm, like the "Fire and Brimstone Coming Doooown ... ."

I tried to stay with Mississippi John Hurt, tried to stick to Big Joe

Turner, but it seemed like all the CDs and albums in the studio shouted, "Live from Tipitina's," "Live from Louisiana," "Live from Lafayette," "Live, Live, Live!" What could I do?

After the show ended at midnight, I stepped knee deep into blue snow and silence sighed. "Jacque-a-Mo-Fi-Na-Nay," I hummed to myself—what does that mean? The aurora borealis dusted the 1:00 A.M. sky as I crunched down the steps, and took care over the sidewalk. Mardi Gras Indian chants tangled in my hair—I crossed the icy street and cut through ice fog, almost home.

"You must have put Voodoo on me..."

I applied and came in second place for two different jobs that I really didn't want; no job, no job, no job! When the year thawed, I bought a brown Isuzu truck and drove across the continent. I was sucked into the oven heat. I would some day stand in a park on the corner of Magazine and Napoleon Avenue and the Nevilles would be right there on the stage, storming and blowing and calling to me, throbs of music pounding my chest.

And standing there before the roar of horns and drums, before the rush of music and rhythm, I would flash back to the basement of the KUAC studio and forward to the steaming uptown park, back into the basement, back to the park, and I would feel dizzy in call and response. I push and pull, shuffle between ice fog and a dripping sauna, my body shakes, my head dizzies, my mind goes weak with recognition like ringworm itch beneath my skin. I spin into melodic joy; I sweat and collapse as the sun sets and the full moon rises yellow and huge, reclaiming me.

Kissing in the Snow

I saw my first Zydeco Band in Fairbanks, Alaska. That night I found hope that a man could love a woman with HIV. My date Shawn and I shook our heads side to side, rock 'n roll style to the Zydeco beat. Shawn danced with a kind of a torso-twisting motion, and I moved more through the hips, but neither of us knew how to Zydeco dance or even two-step.

When Zydeco Express eased into a waltz, I turned towards our seats.

"Hey." Shawn caught my arm. "Don't know why people sit down like that when a slow one starts. Don't have to be star-crossed lovers to slow dance," he said. We danced gently and he held my right hand against his chest. "Hey, we're doin' alright, Melnick," he whispered in my ear. He called all of his friends by last name, and it sounded surprisingly affectionate when he said mine. We walked home afterwards through fresh snow. I wondered if I would soon have occasion to tell Shawn about the HIV, if I should before we kissed. I wondered how he would respond.

I first met Shawn at the graduate Creative Writing students' meeting. It was my second year at the University of Alaska in Fairbanks. Since my HIV diagnosis, I was afraid to live overseas, as originally planned. But Alaska seemed exciting with jagged mountains of snow, wolves, moose and the Auroras Borealis. That afternoon, I felt good, casually dressed in my overalls and a tank top, my hair braided into two neat pigtails.

"Hi, I'm Shawn," said a young man with a full brown beard, his voice heavy with a Massachusetts accent as he shook my hand. I was unimpressed by this plain-faced, pale-skinned man.

We ended up working in the Writing Center together at night, and during those first quiet fluorescent-lit evenings, Shawn asked me for feedback on a story he was working on. The following week, he confided in me, telling me about a step brother who had recently died. I didn't think we were that close. Afterwards, we walked to the Blue Marlin, a dark, log cabin building and favorite pizza establishment and we became friends, sharing pizza many late nights.

***

A few nights later, Shawn and I went out to hear Willis Prudhomme and Zydeco Express, a band from Louisiana. We speculated as to how a Louisiana band happened to come to Fairbanks, Alaska in the dead of winter. Shawn suggested that the band members got really drunk one night after a gig in a Lafayette dance hall and someone said, "Hey, let's go to Alaska!"

I continued the fantasy: "Yeah, Alaska!" the rubboard player shouted. Before they knew it their manager had booked six tickets to Fairbanks and they found themselves stepping from the alligator-swarmed swamps of the Atchafalaya into frigid air and three feet of hard-packed snow.

"Hey, what is this shit!" They all sobered up quickly.

***

Sitting in my tiny, ugly, wood-panel walled apartment we listened to CDs. I played Tracy Chapman's *Fast Cars* and Shawn pretended to like it a lot. We sat on my small couch, in our wool socks, our Sorrell snow boots parked by the door. His arm around my shoulders, we talked about his travels in Africa, and my two years in the Central African Republic. Shawn had taken an overland truck tour across the continent from North to South. I laid on the couch and he traced his truck journey with an international crew of Europeans across my stomach. It sounded like a kind of rustic, European party cruise on wheels with African scenery rolling by.

"Gotta' tell you something," I said.

"Okay, tell me," he said, his hazel eyes half-closed like a content lynx.

Tracy Chapman sang. She played simple guitar chords, bluesy.

The refrigerator buzzed. I thought of the muted headlights through the ice fog on University Avenue. The baseboard heater crackled and creaked.

"Love this refrain," I said.

"Me too," Shawn pulled me closer, opened his cat eyes.

Chapman's voice sang low, like the resonating hums of the heavy cargo trucks running along the Alaskan highways. Honest and dark. Then her voice cried upward, released a wail.

"I have HIV," I blurted out. I rambled on about Africa, a lover, the cyst on my ovary, condoms and HIV. I watched his eyes, waited for rejection, unspoken assumptions about who I slept with, my diseased self, my danger to him, I waited for judgments.

Shawn's face remained passive, but his eyes grew wide.

"You might want to think about this," I said.

"Hey," he said, "I'm not going anywhere. I'm still here, aren't I? I'm not running away."

we gotta make a decision...or we could die this way

Chapman's voice cut through the dim light. Dry air sucked moisture out of our skin, from our lips, from our mouths. I felt the static in our clothes from the dry, brittle cabin air.

***

Shawn and I stood knee-deep in snow, kissing as stars pulsed above. Every week after we left the Writing Center, Shawn walked me to the steps that led down the campus hill. We began to spend nights at my apartment, and a year later we moved into an apartment together. Unexpectedly, I had a boyfriend. I liked him. He was clever, playful, quirky. I no longer saw him as ordinary looking, but handsome with clear, hazel lynx eyes. I liked his boyish face and smooth, broad shoulders.

We never made love because Shawn was too afraid, even with a condom. I was disappointed. But he was the best boyfriend possible, I assumed. During our two years together, Shawn's fears boiled inside him like a pot of mushy pasta.

We rode mountain bikes together over ice and snow-crusted sidewalks, to go to the only shopping mall in town. We wore matching, dark-mirrored sun glasses against the blinding glare of the noon sun on freshly fallen snows. We ate lots of pizza at the Blue Marlin and went to the lousy movies that came to town. He read my essays about Africa and I read his short stories. He said I needed to research and include more historical and political information to reveal people's social conditions. He admired the travel writings of Paul Theroux and valued a political focus with a cynical edge. I told Shawn that he needed to use more personal information and that making broad political statements after driving across a continent with a truck full of drunk Europeans wasn't enough; he needed to speak to individuals who lived there. We ate eggs and bacon for breakfast, I cooked spaghetti from scratch; he micro-waved hotdogs and served them with a sprig of parsley on the side and we laughed. We listened to Shawn's REM, Eurythmics, Bruce Springstein and CARS CDs. We listened to my Stevie Wonder, Bobby McFerrin, and Roberta Flack CDs. As the sun set at 2:00 p.m. over the deep rolls of blue-hued snow outside our window, we danced in the living room in our flannel shirts and wool socks; we danced with static-wild hair. In the cave of deepest winter, November, December, January, February, we awoke with the 10:30 a.m. sunrise, drank tea and watched watercolor shadows of pink and blue run over the fresh surface of old snow.

***

In the spring, I went to my doctor in Fairbanks and the nurse struggled to draw my blood. I knew there would be trouble when she hesitated, then wrapped the rubber strap around my right upper arm too tightly—it hurt. She took too long and tentatively touched her finger into the crook of my arm in search of a throbbing blue vein. Her small hands trembled; she jabbed too cautiously and no blood came. Then she jabbed too hard, but still no blood flow. She apologized as she tried the left arm and she wrapped the rubber strap too tightly again. She said she was sorry again; sorry when not enough blood came; sorry when she had to begin again; sorry as she asked for help from the doctor. About a week later, a blue, quarter-sized lump appeared on the inside of my elbow and it remained for over a month. I was surprised years later, when I moved to New Orleans, that phlebotomists drew my blood easily, causing little pain.

My doctor gave me the results of my blood labs in her office. This was the first time my t-cells had been tested since I was diagnosed two years before. In those two years my t-cells had fallen from 800 to 400. Normal is between 700 and 1000.

Instead of taking the bus home from the hospital, I walked 40 minutes home, inhaling crisp spring air, and my watery eyes were like kaleidoscopes that broke the brilliant sunlit snow into glittering prisms of blue sky and blurry clusters of suns. When I got home, I collapsed onto the bed and closed my eyes. I wondered if this was the beginning of falling t-cells until I became ill and died. Shawn came home a couple hours later and I told him about the results. He sighed as he lay by my side and put his arms around me. "It's hopeless," he said, his lips a breath away from mine. I did not want Shawn to fall into the hole of despair with me—I wished he would reach in a hand to pull me out. My hope slowed then froze.

***

I had recently discovered the Nevilles Brothers CD, *Yellow Moon*. I turned the volume up loud, danced around the living room. I loved the heavy conga drum rhythms and cool harmonies.

"Down, please," Shawn said. He was reading.

I motioned him to come dance with me, but he wouldn't. I turned the music down, but kept moving my hips, closed my eyes, pretended I was dancing at the edge of the Bayou. I would be graduating at the end of the next academic year and I had a fantasy of buying a truck and driving south to New Orleans. I imagined music in dark, smoky little clubs with rickety bar stools and crowded, sweaty dance floors. If there was so much music, surely cover charges would be low, and with writing as my passion, I never expected to make much money.

"You wish you were black," I heard Shawn's voice.

I opened my eyes. "No." I felt a sting. "I like what I am, it's about music," I said.

Shawn looked back down at his book. I went and sat down in the kitchen, studied the photo of the Nevilles on the back of the CD. The drums pounded on "Wake Up." I could almost feel the deep voices swell inside my chest like a thawing spring river. I wondered if I wished I was black. I didn't think so. I second-guessed myself, wondered if he was right. Why did he say that?

I was beginning to outlive my projected life span, and I wanted more. I lay beside Shawn each night skin to skin, each of us wrapped up in our separate webs of frustration. I squirmed in my cocoon.

***

I began to dig a bed for a spring garden. Everything grew quickly in the long days of summer, and seedlings exploded along with the weeds. I sunk a shovel into the ground and turned the soil. Shawn saw me through our large picture window next to the kitchen table. He winked at me, then came outside, took the shovel, lifted and turned the earth easily, for me. He loved me, I knew this. I loved him too.

"A little garden's nothing," Shawn said.

I reached down to pull the weeds between turns.

"Used to do this for a living," he said.

"I know," I said, recalling his stories of working for a landscaping company.

"Would never do this kind of thing again," he said. "A shitty job." Shawn lowered his voice and I moved closer to hear. "Nigger work," he said.

I felt that sting again. My mind flashed to thoughts of Africa. I saw Awa Hamat's shining smile, her wide 16-year-old eyes, her skin as black as new velvet. She and her sisters stroked my head, made me sweet tea with cloves. These friends still sent me letters on thin sheets of airmail paper, lit with colorful stamps and these friends were part of my experience, a part of me. Then I thought of accusations in the past that I am self-righteous. Maybe. But a bottom-feeder feeling twisted in the mud bottom of my stomach.

Shawn dug down into the garden and I watched filthy, snow-silt coated cars rumble along University Avenue.

"Breakfast?" Shawn asked.

"Not hungry," I said.

Shawn shrugged.

***

On the night after I returned from a job interview in Barrow, Alaska, I felt a tingling sensation on my brow. I had been invited to a party that night, but skipped it to try to sleep off a clinging headache. Shawn rode to the party with my friend Suzanne. I took a couple aspirin and went to bed. I woke up at about eleven p.m. and noticed another bump on my eyelid, another near my eyebrow and the needle-pain persisted. My headache had intensified, and I felt nauseated and frightened. I wondered if these were first signs of AIDS. I called the host of the party and asked for Suzanne. I asked her to take me to the hospital.

"No problem, Trece," she said. The lack of panic in her voice calmed me. Shawn and Suzanne brought me to the hospital in Suzanne's Jeep, and several hours later I was diagnosed with shingles. The doctor gave me five medications that all had separate schedules, but I could barely understand what he was saying, I felt so sick. I went home, took the first pills, then slept hard.

Shawn wrote down my medications on a clipboard and came into the room periodically with a glass of water and my next scheduled pills, or with soup, or just to talk to me and hold my hand. I appreciated his gentle care. But even in my fog, I could sense his alarm at the line of sores that crossed my brow. I had been told that shingles follow lines of nerves, and I spent days with headaches, and a jellyfish stinging pain clung to my forehead. My eye ached and the dotted line of sores made me feel nauseous.

I healed within two weeks and returned to classes and to work in the Writing Center. Shawn no longer kissed me on the lips and he became more hesitant to touch me. I was hurt and felt so diseased.

***

Shawn walked into the Writing Center with a smile on his face. He

98

kissed me on the cheek and I glanced around to see if anyone saw.

"Melnick," he said as he squatted next to me. "Got test results, it's negative!" he whispered. He had been tested for HIV the week before.

I felt glad that he was negative, but sad that he assumed he was really at risk. Shawn got tested for HIV periodically. Even after we were no longer kissing, were just sleeping side by side, he would get tested, then come to me relieved that the test had come out negative. I would never wish otherwise, but how would he get it? We barely touched. He kept thinking of the shingles, the sores that had appeared across my forehead. His fears ate at him and the more he tested, the more his apprehension grew.

***

"I'm so afraid," Shawn said as he lay close to me on the couch.

I put my arms around him and let him talk.

"I'm sorry," he said.

I suggested that we talk with a counselor, but he insisted that no one should know. I wondered if I was an embarrassment to him. I had joined a support group, and sometimes he would come along to support me, but never for himself. He felt he didn't need it. I was the one with the problem. It bothered me that he did little research, and refused to talk to anyone about it. His fears burned inside of him like a house fire swallowing papers and books and sticks of furniture, as flames sparked and spat.

***

I knew I didn't want to keep in touch with Shawn after I left Alaska. I also realized that I didn't want a future sleeping next to a man who did not want to learn more about HIV, who feared me, who could sigh and say, "It's hopeless." In my gut, I knew that I would rather be alone than dragged down further into despair. And Shawn admitted that a part of him felt relieved that I was leaving because the relationship was stressful for him.

I made tentative decisions about my future. I knew that I did not want to feel even a subtle undercurrent of racism from a lover. I did not want to be with a man who might pull me away from other people I cared about. I would rather be alone than with a man who did not believe in my future. My life was returning to me.

HARMLESS

I HAD ENTERED THE VAST EMPTY SPACES of the west between New Mexico and Texas, an area where the radio will not pick up any music and if you hit the scan button it will just scan the radio station void until you turn it off. I drove from Alaska to Louisiana after graduate school. Since I was on the highway that runs along the old Route 66, I put in an *Asleep at the Wheel* tape and waited for the song Route 66 to come on so I could sing along about driving through, "Sain't Looey," Joplin, Oklahoma City, Amarillo and Gallup, New Mexico.

Hours later, just as "Don't Ask Me (Why I'm Going to Texas)" came on, I noticed a lanky young guy standing on the shoulder of Interstate 45. I was west of Tucumcari and the man held up a hand lettered cardboard sign that said, "HARMLESS." I wondered if I should give him a ride. I thought of highway rapes and murders and didn't like the idea of picking up a man who is likely to be much stronger than I. He might have a gun or knife. I got off the interstate and circled back. The sign "HARMLESS" made me chuckle, as though he recognized a female driver's feeling of vulnerability, that he even empathized. He was trying to show that he was not the serial killer of my imagination. Perhaps he really was harmless.

I slowed to a stop and waited as he jogged up to the passenger's side. He had a scruffy beard and a lavender bandana wrapped around his head and knotted in back like a pirate. The young man put his backpack behind the seat and got into the truck. He told me that he was heading back from California on his way home to Boston. He appeared to be young and enjoying an adventure of coast to coast travel.

I dropped him off in Amarillo, a few hours down the road. I would turn south to camp in Palo Duro Canyon.

As I meet men in the clubs of New Orleans, men who ask for my phone number or who offer me theirs, I imagine highways lined with bristle-faced hitch-hikers, all watching me pass by as I try to decide whether or not to slow down, stop by the side of the road and allow the stranger to get into my car. I wonder when I am in danger as I consider the risks. I look for a hand-lettered sign that says, "HARMLESS."

ZACKARY

I WANDERED OVER TO ZACKARY who was standing by the bar. He put an arm around me. I was at Mid-City Rock'n'Bowl in New Orleans, where I went most Thursday nights. I enjoyed dancing—though I was just learning—and it was fun to flirt with the men I had met.

"I almost called you this week," I said.

"How?" he asked. "You don't have my number"

"I looked it up in the phone book, you live on Octavia Street," I said.

"You rascal, you," he said with a grin. "That would have been alright."

I met Zackary a couple of months earlier. I had admired how Zackary danced, the way he spun on long legs, then halted suddenly in place, and continued on beat. He always danced so close to his partners, usually a petite, red-haired woman who spun with him, and he always looked hard into her eyes with each move. I wanted to dance with him, but was so clumsy. I didn't understand his steps as I watched him move quickly and smoothly across the floor with his graceful partner.

Zach asked where I worked and I named the university.

"What subject?" he drawled.

"Creative writing," I said, and he asked me what kind of writing I did, if I had been published, if I had a book published, if I had a manuscript, and I was taken aback by his interest—no one I had met at this club or in the dance scene had shown much interest in writing. He opened up conversation on creative non-fiction, what it really was, whether it was irresponsible journalism. I tried to turn conversation towards him and he said he worked at Tulane but was vague about the work, said it wasn't important like the job I do. I felt embarrassed, wondered if I appeared arrogant.

I danced with Zackary again and he held me around the waist, close, and looked into my eyes with a smile. I looked away, looked at him back and forth, not sure how to meet his gaze as he stepped across the dance floor and when he spun us around, two, three, four times, it was like flying, my feet lifting off the floor briefly at times, and the sudden stop felt like a soft fall, and the stepping across the floor continued, as I tried to follow, uncomfortable with Zackary's blue-fire gaze.

We flew in circles like courting crows. He again asked me about that creative nonfiction, teasing. "You don't mind if I fuck with you, do you?" he asked.

"Not if you don't mind me fucking back with you," I said, but regretted my choice of words the moment they came out.

"Oooh, I like the sound of that," Zackary said, studying my face as a blush burned across my skin.

He waltzed with me with long, fast steps and I lost the rhythm.

"I can tell you're thinking too hard, trying too hard," Zackary said.

I felt his tongue in my ear and pulled away, though the music moved my feet in time and my pulse raced.

After the band stopped, Zackary asked if I wanted to get donuts later. "Let's take your car," he said, "since I don't have one."

By doughnuts, he meant beignets. It was 2:00 a.m., my favorite time to go to Café du Monde when the crowd tends to be low key. We drove to the French Quarter, to Cafe Du Monde. The air was warm, breezing through the tables, and a Vietnamese waitress took our order for beignets, coffee for Zackary, hot chocolate for me. Zackary took off his hat, and for the first time I saw the long strands of hair combed straight back from his receding hairline. Sweaty head, sweaty hair—but he still looked handsome.

"You should have said you don't drink coffee," Zackary said.

"I knew I'd find something I like." Our legs and knees barely touched beneath the table.

I told Zackary about my breakup with the most recent boyfriend, about deciding to learn to Zydeco, about my family. He had been married once.

"Did you like being married?" I asked.

"Yes, I did," he said, and I liked the certain honesty of his answer.

I told him I wanted to marry some day and that I was thirty-seven.

"I'm a lot older than that," he said.

At the table just behind us slumped a street performer dressed in gold polyester with face painted gold. He sipped coffee and stared.

"How old?" I asked.

But he wouldn't tell me and I wondered—forties or fifties?

He told me of spending many years in California where he went to become a monk, but changed his mind and began to study martial arts. He talked about learning to Zydeco dance on his return to New Orleans, about intense practice alone, with a shirt in his arms to be comfortable holding a woman, a point I found hard to believe remembering how when we danced, he playfully knocked his knee between my legs on the floor, how he had stuck his tongue in my ear to get me loosen up, he said. He complained about people coming for the wrong reasons, to pick someone up, saying that this attitude was harming the quality of dancing. Yet I felt he was trying to pick me up.

Zackary told me about work being done on in his apartment after recent floods. He commented on lazy workers who went through his boxes.

"Why?" I asked. "Why would they do such a thing?"

A young woman wearing a short black dress and heels sat at the table with the gold street performer and I wondered how they knew each other.

"I don't know why they did that," he said. "—Well, yes I do."

He looked downward to the left at two head-bobbing pigeons as though they would have the answer.

"I have some controversial materials," he said.

At a table behind us, three long-limbed teen boys leaned close together whispering. I looked back at Zachary and asked with my eyes, *What kinds of materials might those be?*

"Books on alternative sex," he said.

Pigeons picked at discarded beignet crumbs. I wondered if Zackary was gay. Maybe into group sex or Rocky Horror costumes.

"Books on sadomasochism, a gun—they were probably looking though the books and laughing." And then Zackary continued talking about his frustration with the landlord, his refusal to return phone calls promptly. Pigeons tugged at mutilated beignets between tables.

I stared at him. My knees withdrew from his. Zackary continued to talk around what he had just said and I imagined a naked couple beating each other with whips, in a rumpled bed. My horror filled the space between us.

"No!" Zackary said, his voice hard and sudden, as though he had seen the picture in my mind. "I don't tie up young women and torture them!"

"Then I'm safe having you in the car with me?"

"Yes, but that's alright, I can take the street car home!"

"No, I'll take you," I said.

He was fuming, I was shaking. Torn beignets lay on our plates. We walked out together, but Zachary stalked in the opposite direction to catch the St. Charles streetcar.

***

The next week, when I went to Rock n' Bowl, I saw Zachary, but pretended I did not. This time, I didn't wonder if I might meet any nice men—I only wanted to dance. And I felt happier than ever, dancing with a rhythmic freedom I felt for the first time as I swayed in one man's arms, spun around the floor with another and we swung together—apart. Another slow zydeco waltz. This time I realized I had come to be close to the dance, close to the music, to be close to myself.

Intimacy

I WAS SINGLE. IN MY WORLD, if I was not dating there seemed little occasion for touch, a hug, a kiss or holding hands, and my family members lived hundreds of miles away. Also, HIV made dating problematic and sometimes left me feeling alone.

Driven by my desire to be touched, I decided to learn how to Zydeco dance. As with other dance styles for couples, the man holds his arm around the woman's waist, she has her hand on his shoulder, and partners clasp hands. People tend to dance Zydeco very close, legs between legs, practically groin to groin.

***

When I lived in the Central African Republic, well before I came in contact with HIV, I went to the French doctor's house one afternoon to pick up mail for myself and the other Peace Corps volunteers in my town of Bangassou. He had been nice enough to bring the mail back for us from Bangui, the capital city. Like the others, I was eager for letters from my parents and friends.

As I approached the house, I saw a black chimpanzee with a rope around her waist, tied to a tree. The forty-five-pound primate began shrieking at me, baring her teeth as she bounced up and down, straining at the rope. She frightened me—I had never seen chimpanzees up close. I had only seen them behind bars in zoos, wearing ballerina skirts at the circus, or swinging through the trees on *National Geographic* TV specials.

Cautious, but curious, I inched closer. I admired the agile, long-fingered hands and the deep brown eyes as she howled her primate threats. I imagined how the sharp incisors could bite into my flesh, how the shrieking jaws could clamp down on my leg. I edged closer to the wailing animal and then she leapt at me, and in a flashing instant her legs and arms wrapped around my waist and neck, quick as a boa constrictor wraps coils around its squirming meal. My body froze and my heart pounded as hairy, warm limbs squeezed me. Then I felt the chimp lie her head on my shoulder like a human child, fallen silent. Her screeches were not threats but cries—this baby just wanted her mother.

I stroked the fur on her back and her quick breathing began to slow. Then she lifted her head off my shoulder to look me in the eye and I ached at her urgent need for affection. I stepped closer to the tree so the rope wouldn't pull on the chimp's waist, and I lowered myself to the ground to sit cross-legged. As I embraced her, I wondered if this baby was found or stolen, and if a hunter had shot the mother. Dirt-covered bits of mango and banana lay nearby and there was a shallow bowl of water a few feet away. But all she wanted at that moment was to be held. Her soft eyes said, "Please don't put me down, ever." When I had to unwrap her arms to leave, she stared at me as though I had deceived her.

The sepia eyes of this chimpanzee have haunted me ever since. And sometimes I too feel that bottomless need, feel like screeching and throwing my arms around someone, anyone.

***

I have always loved the bluesy wailing of the Zydeco accordion, and the invigorating rubboard rhythms. My legs thought they could dance to the music, but I didn't know how. I decided it was time to overcome this hurdle and I also hoped to meet eligible bachelors. But at least I would have a chance to move to this music, and to be touched by men.

Beau Jocque and the Zydeco Rollers were playing at Mid-City Rock 'n' Bowl on the Thursday night I went dancing, Zydeco night. I walked up the steps of the long turquoise hallway, and stepped through the archway that was graced by a faded print of the Virgin Mary. As I entered the club, I could feel the bass sounds beat deep in my chest as Beau Jocque's voice boomed. One side of the open room was filled with bowling lanes. Nestled at the far end of the room was the stage where the band played. Above the dance floor, a spinning disco ball scattered spots of light over the frenzied mass of dancers.

I sat by myself in a corner and studied the couples' steps. They stepped and pranced in cowboy boots but it looked to me as if each couple were doing a completely different move. Some dancers stood apart, kicking forward, grabbing hands and then spinning around. Others just leaned into each other and swayed from side to side, knees between knees. I couldn't follow the steps, but I moved my hips to the rhythm, half-hoping someone would ask me to dance. Beyond the dance floor, I could see people cradling blue-flecked bowling balls. Each of the bowlers would run, slide, release the ball and then break into dance as it wobbled down the lopsided lanes toward the pins.

I walked over to the bar for a coke and waited to be served by one of the smooth-faced bar maids, all clad in pleated turquoise and black bowling skirts. Over the bar hung a Heineken Beer sign with a neon-lit orange and green accordion-playing alligator. As I leaned against the bar, I felt the floor tremble beneath the pummel of the heavy-heeled dancers.

"Would you like to dance?" asked a tall, handsome, pecan-brown man. He wore a white cowboy hat, blue jeans and brown leather boots. He had close-cropped hair, was lean, and looked to be in his late forties, about fifteen years older than I. He wore rectangular glasses over his Cherokee nose and freckled high cheek bones. The gentleman called himself "Bogart" and he led me to an open, out-of-the-way area between the dance floor and the bar. He stood beside me to show me the steps, a couple of quick side steps, then a leaning back-step move. Bogart took my right hand in his left and put an arm around my waist to guide me. His skin smelled like lemons.

I liked Bogart's easy movements, not wild or competitive as with some of the other dancers. He had an intelligent gaze and gentle demeanor, but I didn't like how close he held me, or the way he glanced down at my chest and gave me sly smiles. His wedding band gleamed on his finger as I tolerated his occasional suggestive comments.

Even after several weeks of practice, I would still lose the rhythm.

I panicked and struggled to find the beat again.

"Maybe I should take a Zydeco class," I said.

As Bogart turned me gently, I scanned the strands of green, purple and gold Mardi Gras-Christmas lights that ran the length of the room.

Give him corn bread, Beau Jocque's bass voice sang.

What you need lessons for?" Bogart said, momentarily taking his eyes off my cleavage.

"So I can learn better," I said.

"You don't need lessons," Bogart said, "I'm teachin' you."

"I've never been good at this," I said, "I think it would give me more confidence."

"You can just pay me that money, if that'll give you more confidence," his eyes played mischievously. "I can write you up a bill right now, if ya' want."

The quick rattle-rhythms of the rubboard filled my ears and my feet pounded the floor instinctively.

"Forget it," I laughed.

Rolling bowling balls echoed in the dance hall, punctuated by the clinking of toppled pins.

Tell-me-tell-me-tell-me-right nooooow… I felt my body lean back with the drawn out call of the accordion.

"*Eh Toi!*" Bogart called out as he spun me around on the last notes of the song.

***

In September, I went to the Zydeco Festival in Plaissance, Louisiana. This three day festival takes place on a farm approximately three hours northwest of New Orleans, and features many bands. I arrived at about 3:00 p.m. while the sun was still blazing. Crowds of Zydeco dancers were kicking up red dust as they sweated to the music of Boozoo Chavis. I came alone but soon ran into Bogart. After the sun sank low, we danced in the crowd before the stage and my feet hop-stepped easily. By late evening, my legs ached from hours of stomp-stepping and turning to the music but we kept on dancing.

"I better head home before long," I said.

"Can I come?" Bogart had asked me this before.

"Think your wife might miss you," I said.

"Maybe," he said.

"If she doesn't, you're probably doing something wrong," I said, "and then I wouldn't have much use for you either."

"Maybe you could give me some pointers." He raised one eyebrow.

"Yeah, right," I said. "I'm gonna to go get something to eat."

I needed to take my pills; they had to be taken with food. Along the perimeter of the grounds, food stands advertised fried softshell crab po-boys, barbequed pork sandwiches, cochon au lait, jambalaya, crawfish etouffe, barbequed ribs and fried catfish. My stomach growled.

"I'll go with you," Bogart said.

I settled on a barbequed pork sandwich. Bogart bought me a coke, got himself a bottle of water, and we sat on a bench that was off to the side, in the shadows.

I reached into the back pocket of my jeans and pulled out my pill box. I placed my sandwich and coke on the bench beside me, opened the little square pill container, and dumped all ten pills out into the palm of my hand.

I left my hand open.

I wanted Bogart to see, wanted to tell him that I had HIV, so that this kind but married man would back off.

"Those vitamins?" Bogart asked.

"Nope, not vitamins," I answered as I popped a couple pills in my mouth and took a swig of Coke. I unwrapped the foil of the pork sandwich and took a bite to kill the bitter taste of the pills.

"You got a cold or something?" he asked.

"No," I said as I swallowed. "I have HIV." I waited for a look of awe.

"Oh, I see," he said. His eyes did not widen. He barely looked up. His tone was flat as though all I had said was that my left foot was slightly larger than my right. I figured he was just good at hiding his emotions, his surprise.

"So does my son," Bogart said, his voice low.

"Oh." This time it was *I* who was surprised. I chewed the dry pork sandwich.

Pleasant breezes cooled my shoulders as Bogart told me about his son, a gay man who was just a couple years younger than I. He was healthy, though he took no medications, and had lived with HIV for nine years.

"*Why-do-you-do-me-like-you-do?*" Zydeco Joe sang in the distance, and then a high-pitched guitar solo stirred the air. I finished my sandwich and we walked back to the center of the field to listen to the band.

***

Bogart was getting a drink, so I took a seat next to him at Rock 'n' Bowl. It had been a week since the Zydeco Festival. Geno Delafose and French Boogie were playing that night.

"Hummm, nice shirt," Bogart said, glancing down.

I ignored the comment.

"How ya' feelin?" he asked. I knew he really wanted to know. I told him that I was fine and he told me that his son was well. Geno Delafose began playing, "*Bon Soir Moreau*," so Bogart pulled me into a close waltz. As we glided around the dance floor, we looked over each other's shoulders, kept watch for sepia shadows of fear. I held onto my friend, felt his hand gently tapping, keeping time on my back; and my screeching primate ache for affection diminished. I closed my eyes, and felt the music rush through me, felt the rubboard rhythms resonate inside, and then the accordion began to wail. I heard it inhale, exhale, inhale.

Support Group

Years ago, a co-worker of mine said that if you gathered a group of friends around a table, and each individual placed her problems in the center of the table and took someone else's in exchange, most people would take back their own burdens.

We were all women in this office and we often discussed our personal lives. I thought about paraplegics, parents of terminally ill children, individuals trailed with a history of abuse as children, families with a suicidal family member. I would be hard-pressed to say that I would exchange my HIV diagnosis for someone else's problems. I can't imagine anyone exchanging her problems for HIV. People adjust to their situations: Louisianans live with hurricane threats and Californians expect earthquakes. We own pain like emotional real estate and it contributes to our identities. Would you exchange your problems for mine? People live most comfortably with the burdens they know best and fear the unfamiliar ones.

***

"There is nothing in the world worse than *this*," said Jason at a meeting of the NO/AIDS Task Force for straight people with HIV. This meeting included three men and two women, including me. Jason told us that he had dated a woman, then found out that she was bisexual, so he decided break up with her. But he admitted that he was relieved to have a reason to reject her. That way, he would not have to tell her that he was HIV positive and risk being rejected by her.

I had joined this group in hopes of discussing dating with HIV. I wanted to explore issues with others, such as when to disclose one's diagnosis. I hoped to learn strategies for negotiating such a conversation.

We could discuss the risks of telling too soon or too late. How does one respond to his lover's fears? But group discussions went in different directions from what I had expected.

"The world *hates* us," Marcus agreed with Jason. Marcus looked to be in his early fifties, silver hair carefully feathered back, blue eyes encircled by gold-rimmed glasses. He was pale-skinned, his face awash in freckles and creases. He wore a bright, tropical shirt and I imagined him wandering through a lush jungle as he fixated on his situation. "I am fine alone," he said. "I don't need anyone." He said he hated people, hated their prejudices, hated what they stood for. I wondered if he meant only prejudices against people with HIV, or if he meant in general. Perhaps Jason and Marcus felt greater frustration in part because they were men, who, according to societal norms, must learn to appear stoic, private. None of the men in the group spoke of friends in whom they confided. They may have lacked a support system, the role I supposed our group was supposed to play.

"Do you think we can get more people in the group?" Marcus asked. "Where can we find more *women* for the group?" He was a bull pawing the ground, ready to charge after the first acceptable cow he saw. He seemed to view the session as an HIV positive swingles meeting. "There's no point in talking to someone who doesn't have it," he said. "They could never understand."

I couldn't tell how old Jason was. He found out that he was HIV positive after becoming very ill, but with a regimen of antiviral drugs, he regained his health. I didn't know if he had shaved his head for style or was bald from age or medical treatment. He looked haggard, which could have been from illness or age. He had tired brown eyes and spoke with a taffy-chewing-slow Southern drawl and muffled voice.

All of the men in the group said they wouldn't consider dating anyone who was not HIV positive because the frustration and pain of having to share information was simply too great. I crossed my arms and legs, leaned back and listened. I felt under inspection, as I sat across the room in one of those ugly, sink-down counseling chairs that are supposed to inspire honest talk. I couldn't imagine dating an angry man.

"Patrice, do you have any HIV positive female friends you could invite?" Marcus asked.

"No, I don't have any," I said. I wondered why I didn't.

Marcus was clad in stylish jeans as he tried to sit upright in a too-soft chair. Jason's arms sprawled across the back of a fake leather couch. Both eager and needy. The room was too small, the ceiling too low, the room warm as a summer bog.

After he found out that he had HIV, Marcus decided to isolate himself. He lived on an island in the Pacific for ten years, said that he was too afraid to be around people. But many years later, he was ready to meet women; he said he had been looking at dating websites for straight people with HIV. The concept surprised me, the thought of searching for a mate with the same affliction.

If I met someone who happened to have HIV, whom I liked very much because, say, we were both crazy about the Talking Heads or we both loved to Zydeco dance or if the guy had a great sense of humor, then maybe both of us having HIV would solidify the bond. But to gravitate towards each other based on a disease, a virus, would almost be like allowing the condition to eclipse other aspects of our identities. I would be concerned that with HIV as our bond, this condition would remain the center of our lives and the negative might overshadow the positive and keep us from enjoying the sparkling futures that were taken away from us, then returned.

If people decided to date others with like conditions, we would need to start more social clubs for people with HIV. Sororities and fraternities for single cancer survivors. People with really bad acne or swingles with athlete's foot or loose knee caps can meet and date others with the same condition. People with chronic allergies date others with allergies, because no one else in the world can understand what that feels like. I realize that HIV is not hay fever. It is life threatening and unique—no one else knows what it feels like to have this condition. But there are many ways to relate. Most people feel the pull of their mortality sooner or later.

***

"There is nothing in the world worse than having HIV," Jason agreed with Marcus. I believed that at one time, too. I asked Jason if he didn't feel grateful to be alive. No, he answered, he did not feel that way. I wondered if he was glad to be alive before he had HIV.

A slender, blond, sad-eyed woman described the first time she found out that she had HIV. She said that at the time she loathed her job and a love relationship was coming to an end, so she found her diagnosis, the promise of death, convenient. A heavyset, bearded man with a clear, soft voice admitted that he had a death wish even before he had HIV. Perhaps because they were not happy before they had HIV, they grew more angry and frustrated after diagnosis. HIV had simply magnified their problems. It seems to me that HIV doesn't change a person; it makes one a more intense version of himself. The sad become sadder.

***

Mortality rattles in my pocket like a little box of pills. I watch my t-cells and viral load rise and fall. I follow the levels like a nervous gambler watches horses race around a track, like a hyped-up Wall Street executive studies his stocks and bonds, fearing a crash. And yet, somehow, if I could lay my burdens on the table, exchange them for yours, I doubt I would. You, hauling your fears in a sack upon your back, you probably wouldn't trade yours for mine, either. Would you?

Writer's Body

I have been startled by the sight of my own body.

As a girl, I was disgusted by the drawings of women in the Superman comic books, women with huge, accentuated breasts and tiny waists. I dismissed the grotesque drawings as overt expressions of male fantasy—no one really looked like that. Then one day as an adult, I looked into a mirror as I wore a clingy t-shirt and realized that my body resembled those of the cantaloupe breasted, wasp-waisted secretaries and heroines of Superman or Spiderman. I was Wonder Woman, like it or not.

I do not think of myself as a pretty woman. I have a large nose and deep lines crease my face, surround my mouth. My top lip is a little short, so my lips never completely close over my teeth, leaving me with a permanent gawk. And I often have dark shadows under my eyes. I have never worn makeup and am too lazy to start now. My stomach has a slight paunch. My body wears various scars collected from childhood mishaps.

I gather that my body, as opposed to my face, is my best physical asset. I have fairly firm arms, shapely legs, and, most of all, breasts. Despite my average looks, I sometimes feel embarrassed and shy about how overtly my body says *Sex*, whether or not this is on my mind. The breasts attract stares, smiles and the occasional proposition. Over the years, I have struggled to deal with the way my body can attract affection or threats. I like to go to clubs to dance and hear live music. Because I live in sweltering New Orleans, I am likely to wear cool, skimpy clothes, which further draws attention to my body. If a man shows interest, he may be thinking of me as Chicky-poo. I negotiate the attention I receive, attention that is sometimes flattering and sometimes frightening.

117

***

"Patrice," a voice said, and I turned to see Hugo. "How are you?" he asked from beneath thick eyebrows, "I was thinking about you."

I was at Mid-City Rock'n Bowl and I stayed until the end, hoping for more practice dancing.

Hugo was a hulking figure with thick torso and narrow hips.

"Really, what were you thinking?" I asked.

"I was thinking about calling you."

The multifaceted silver disco ball glittered and turned behind him.

"Why didn't you?" I asked.

"Oh, I couldn't find your number, all kinds of papers piled up on my table, just couldn't find your number, you know?"

"Yes, I know," I said. Hugo had asked for my phone number a few weeks before, as we danced to Rock'n Doopsie at the Audubon Zoo Swamp Festival.

"So how's your love life?" A slight smile passed over his chiseled Mayan cheekbones.

"Not so good," I answered.

"Why not so good?" Long black hair hung loose around his muscled shoulders.

I told him I couldn't find the kind of man I was looking for.

"What kind are you looking for?" He took a drink from his beer and scanned the room.

"Honest, consistent, kind, not racist… ," I answered.

"What do you want him to look like? Tall? Thin? Big?"

"Doesn't matter, there's all kinds of good-looking," I said, "but these personality traits are hard to find."

"What race?" Perhaps he wondered if a Hispanic man might interest me.

"Doesn't matter," I said. I wondered if he believed me.

"Dark, light, what do you want him to look like?"

"Really, doesn't matter, there's all kinds of cute. I just want honest, consistent."

"Honest…consistent," Hugo mused. "I'll be honest with you, I'll tell you why I didn't call."

"Okay." I folded my arms and leaned back against the bar.

"I didn't call because I just wanted to have sex with you and you seem like the kind of woman who would expect something more."

The night I spoke with Hugo, I noticed that a chilling October breeze had seeped into the city and I knew that temperatures would soon dip down. I had hoped to find a boyfriend by winter, when damp chills would invade my bones. I thought of how a man radiates all that heat in bed. With a companion, I could postpone turning on my heat a little longer. Of course, I considered the potentially substantial savings on my energy bills which could help to conserve our nation's precious natural resources.

"So, you thought I would expect something more? How did you know this?" I asked.

"Male intuition. But really, I want to make *love* to you."

"So you were doing me a favor by not calling," I said. "Let me tell you something." I leaned closer. "I have HIV." I watched his face.

No reaction. "I'll use a sombrero," he said. "I want to make *love* to you," he continued, as though I had said only that I have acne. "Try, Patrice, have sex with me, but don't have feelings."

Although I do not wish to date men like Hugo—eager, sometimes shallow men—I am glad to find handsome men who are not afraid to touch me. It helps me believe that *even I*, with my ordinary face and terrifying disease, *even I* have the powerful tool of pure, physical, feminine beauty.

"Did you hear me?" I asked.

"I believe you. But I want to make *love* to you. I'll use a condom. Will you try, Patrice? Try not to have feelings."

"Do you ask a lot of women? Do many women accept?" I asked Hugo. "I can't control my feelings," I said.

Hugo had cut through the illusion of wanting to have lunch, a cup of coffee and conversation—he openly requested what he wanted. There was an honesty to his approach.

"Just try not to have feelings," Hugo pleaded.

"I *have* tried. Maybe you could have sex with me and try to *have* feelings."

Hugo shook his head, then handed me a scrap of paper with his phone number scribbled on it. "Just want sex—you got my number."

"Yeah, I've got your number." I slid the scrap into my back pocket.

***

I look for solutions to the boyfriend puzzle. Perhaps a man's education level, personality and eating habits will clue me in on the type who could accept a woman with HIV.

The men who, as a group, have been most accepting of my condition have been the most promiscuous men. The more sexually active the man, the more extensive his knowledge of risks and safe sex practices. He is the man who wishes to keep his independence as he lives a life of one-night stands or relations with detached lovers. He may be unfaithful to his lover or wife; he just wants a little affair on the side. He picks out a physical figure that pleases him and then pursues. He offers slippery, flattering lines. Such a man knows how to look at a woman out of the corner of his heavy-lidded eyes, knows how to brush the back of his hand gently against her shoulder. This man is not afraid of long, open-mouthed kisses with an HIV-positive woman; he knows that the virus is not spread this way.

Such a man will not be surprised that I have HIV; he knows that any person can get it, realizes the falseness of stigmas and stereotypes. He is slower to blame, less likely to carry a superior attitude. The man of the one-night stand may be knowledgeable about sex and STDs, regardless of formal education, regardless of ethnicity or culture or class. He wants Wonder Woman. He knows how to use a condom.

***

I have found colleagues to be especially fearful of my HIV status.

Is it because educated men expect security as they hover beneath the shelter of a healthcare plan, reasonable salary and retirement benefits? An educated man may feel in control of his world, may not expect to meet a female colleague with HIV. One colleague who I dated for about a month called me up one night to explain that he had become more afraid than he expected. I later recalled that he also feared flying, avoided meat for fear of hormones, and worried about radiation from power lines near his house. It seems that the more fears a man harbors, the less likely that he and I will be compatible.

Men who break out in a cold sweat at the thought of flying may well be afraid of me. Vegetarians are not a good bet. Men who fear the hormones in their meat, inorganic irradiated fruits and vegetables or men who avoid dairy products, eggs, meat, fish, chicken—such men inevitably become afraid of getting HIV from me. The nut and berry eaters, the vegans are not good dates, nor are the men who have nightmares about genetically engineered potatoes and corn. Those who worry about antibiotics, pesticides, cancer-causing dioxins, contaminated meat, and processed sugars are likely to fear me. Men who quake at the thought of radiation from power lines, computer screens, cellular telephones, radio and television broadcasts, and microwave communications links are not good bets. Those who fear that the local water supply contains unnatural additives such as chlorine and fluoride would likely tremble upon hearing that I have HIV. Such a man may see me as a walking hazard site.

***

In my mind, handsome comes in a variety of tones. But I have met more white men who are afraid of me than people of color. This aspect seems to overshadow education levels. Men like Hugo tend to be familiar with condom use and are less likely to try to figure out if I am a promiscuous drug user, less likely to apply stigma. Perhaps promiscuous, minority, blue collar carnivores best suit me. I have considered placing an ad in the personals:

"Friendly, spirited, HIV-positive woman looking for kind man for long romantic walks on the beach. Prefer sleeps-with-anything-that-moves, beef-eating, non-white man. Call before weather turns cold."

***

One of my African American students wrote a personal narrative about when he was seventeen years old and two New Orleans policemen pulled him over. One officer slammed him up against the hood of his car and held a gun to his head. The other searched him and ran a check to see if the car he was driving was stolen—it was his mother's. The young man's eyes teared up as he drove away, thinking about the hard shine of the officer's insect-like mirrored sunglasses. I know that many middle-class black teens are used to being followed around in clothing stores by sales clerks who are watching for shoplifters. They know that the color of their skin is often a liability, and that "good" behavior might fail to keep them safe. While a professional white man can build a life in which he feels secure, a dark-skinned man may sense that life is inevitably risky. I wonder if the experience of a man who has been pulled over by hostile policemen at least once in his life is less likely to be alarmed when a friend admits that she has HIV. In a life where a dark complexion carries the stereotype of car thief, shoplifter or HIV carrier, does this person grow more sensitive to the struggles of others who carry stigmas?

***

I have become used to my ordinary face. I expect my Wonder Woman figure to attract different types of men, though the HIV information may flash like a caution light. Or perhaps the hovering man will brush away concerns like a pesky moth. When I speak with a male friend, I like it if he looks me in the eye and strokes my arm with his unafraid hand.

NoLove Condoms
Products for Our Modern World

Enjoy the Moment!

Latex sheathes have protected men and women against pregnancy and sexually transmitted diseases for many years. But now sexually active men and women can utilize protection against infection from that sticky feeling called emotion. Now you can avoid the messy cleanup of one-night-stands. The revolutionary, medically developed and tested NoLove vinyl condoms guard against emotions, with love-blocking amoricides.

If used properly, condoms will help to reduce the risk of transmission of affection, and many other sexually contracted emotions including "wish-he'd-call," "genital-please-her," "congenial-warts," "if-only-she-wasn't-married B and C," "If-only-he-didn't-have-a-criminal-record," and "Wish-it-wasn't-over-so-fast!"

Some individuals may experience a slight irritation to amoricides. If this should happen to you, consult a psychiatrist. No method of contraception can provide 100% protection against pregnant pauses, or sexually transmitted affection.

How to use a NoLove condom:

Handle with care. No Love Condoms can be rendered ineffective if used in conjunction with candle-lit dinners, perfume, or Al Green love songs.

NoLove Extra InSensitive Condoms are super thin to allow physical passion, but tough enough to provide exceptional desensitivity. NoLove

Extra InSensitive Condoms set you free to enjoy the pleasure of sex while being confident that you're protected from Emotional Aftermath (EA).

Warning:
Never use the same condom more than once.
Never use same partner more than once.

REMEMBER:
  • Extra InSensitive
  • Super strong for less feeling
  • Lubricated with amoricides to help desensitize

Available in a variety of sensible colors including:
  Eggshell
  Ivory
  Ecru

Each Package Contains:
11 premium vinyl condoms
Anaesthetized for effectiveness

These packages are tamper evident.
If package is damaged do not use.
If partner is damaged, do not use.

Get the most out of Life!
Desensitize your nights with NoLove Condoms.

Coming Soon: Flush that loving feeling away with After Thought, the Morning After Pill.

Gifts

"Hı," I saıd.

"Hey," Ian said, a broad, smile on his face, as if nothing happened, "Get me a spade," he said, holding up a bag of flower bulbs in his right hand. I found a spade in my shed and handed it to him. He went into the front yard flower bed, bent down in the sun and dug into the earth, planting bulbs, patting the soil down. He planted the tiger lily, daffodil and amaryllis bulbs that his mother had sent to him as a gift the week before. He patted soft dirt over newly planted bulbs and he cultivated forgiveness.

In the first six months that Ian and I dated, we argued often, usually about the status of our relationship. He would typically show affection one day, cooking me dinner and telling me hilarious jokes. Then a day or two later he acted aloof, did not call or return my calls, as though to establish that our involvement was not serious, to preserve his independence. Ian never called to apologize or talk over the situation. Instead, after several days of no contact he would ride his red mountain bike to my house, his only mode of transportation, and knock on my door.

I met Ian a couple of years after I moved to New Orleans. It was the night I had learned that I was hired at my first University job, and I went to Café Istanbul, on Frenchman Street, to celebrate and hear Latin music. Frenchman Street was in a Bohemian part of town where freshly pierced twenty-somethings and older tie-dyed folks loitered outside the clubs and coffee shops. As I stood up close to the stage, a young man came up behind me and asked me to dance. His wide blue eyes looked young and hopeful beneath thinning blond hair. I didn't know how to Salsa dance, but he said he would show me. Incense wafted through the room, mixed with scent of sweat and cologne. Ian danced well, and I barely managed to follow his lead.

After the club closed, the slender young man walked me to my car. I said I had to leave, had for the first time left my dog alone with my new cat. I hoped the cat was okay.

"I wouldn't worry, they probably got your penny jar and are sitting around playing poker 'bout now."

I laughed.

Ian was new in town, had come to New Orleans under the pretense to attend graduate school. He was enrolled at a local University, but I soon realized that he really came to New Orleans to become a Latin jazz musician. He played upright base. Ian and I spent time together as friends a few times. As I was driving him home one night, I found that Ian was only twenty-three, eight years younger than me. I told him that I was thirty one, thinking that he would be surprised and would not attempt to become involved with me. I assumed that such a young man would prefer a younger woman, someone with bright blue eyes and a petite figure. But he was not deterred.

One night I invited Ian over for dinner. I cooked Mexican food. That was the night we became more than friends, and I told him that I had HIV. I told him to take some time to research HIV, to help him decide if he was comfortable seeing a woman with HIV. And I invited him to tell anyone he wanted to, hoping he would learn about it and think things through. I would not enter another sexless relationship with a man, as I had with Shawn in Alaska.

Ian didn't join any support groups and didn't do much research on HIV. But he had a friend who was a physical therapist, a man Ian respected. "Just use a condom. Use it every time," his friend said matter-of-factly. Ian must have been reassured by the casual attitude of this trusted friend with a medical background. Perhaps his fears were calmed because he had someone to talk to, so his emotions did not build up inside the way they had with secretive Shawn. Ian got tested for HIV periodically, and he may have worried some, though he did not share this worry with me.

I wanted to talk everything over, but Ian, like others I'd dated, didn't like to talk. He was a poet through action, creating metaphors everywhere. Plants are love. Ian planted flower bulbs throughout the flower beds and the ground bloomed prides of untamed tiger lilies, clumps of dripping yellow daffodils and explosions of shell-white and crimson amaryllis. After a late spring argument with Ian, he begged me to let him work with me in the yard one afternoon. He trimmed the lower branches of the Japanese magnolia which had grown into a thick of broad green summer leaves and bloomed lilac, cup-shaped flowers every January. He sweated all afternoon, guided his chain saw, snipped shrubs with clippers. We hauled eight-foot stalks of fragrant ginger from the backyard into the front for the garbage man to pick up. At the end of the day, he planted an angels' trumpet plant that he had rooted from a cutting, for me.

***

I came to realize that it was possible to be intimate with a man who would not fear me. I felt relieved that Ian saw me as more than a woman with HIV. We dated for over five years, and I loved being with a musician, the house blasting the songs of Ruben Blades, Carlos Santana, or Tito Puente. Ian adored my dogs, Tomboula and Samba, and took them for long walks through the neighborhood. Like me, he was left handed and liked to draw and I loved watching him play concerts at the local clubs into the early hours of the morning. He was so involved with his music that it was easy for me to take time for myself to concentrate on writing. He told hilarious jokes, was smart, creative, and brought me gifts of music. He grew thick tangles of flowers in the yard. And he was not afraid of me.

But eventually we broke up because I wanted to make our relationship permanent. He was not ready for this step. Years after the separation that left me melancholy, the angels' trumpet grew huge with long, coral hued blossoms that called with sensual aromas. Ian had planted himself into the soil, into my life. Flowers bloomed for years and he would never be completely weeded out of my memory; tender shoots of nostalgia resurfaced unexpectedly on warm, humid spring mornings.

THOUGHTS ON WRITING A MEMOIR AT FORTY

I had a drink with Antoine in a narrow, dark, neon-lit bar in the French Quarter in New Orleans. The jukebox played Dr. John's "Right Place" as I sipped a coke and he drank a beer. He asked me what I was writing, so I told him a memoir.

I had met Antoine while Zydeco dancing at Mid-City Rock 'n Bowl. I found him unattractive, I confess. He was a tall, ungainly man who didn't strike my fancy. But after I had spoken with him on several occasions I found him to be intelligent and interesting. A lawyer who worked for a social rights organization, he defended people on death row, especially minorities who had likely been discriminated against. And he knew a lot about blues music and the little juke joints scattered about in Louisiana, Mississippi and Tennessee. So I accepted his invitation to meet for a drink.

The yellow and blue neon lights in the windows flashed behind Antoine's huge torso and he seemed to be trying to mask his surprise that I was writing a memoir. It never fails; whenever I use the word "memoir," eyebrows are raised.

"Well, I guess on down the road," Antoine tilted his head to the side as though carefully choosing his words, "on down the road you can write the sequel." He looked at me adoringly and his bright blue eyes twinkled. I was touched and amused by his response. He seemed to think me too young to write a memoir; those are written by crusty old men who have survived a couple of wars, at least one economic depression, and years of hunger to better achieve some kind of personal, political or social triumph. These men spend the last years of their lives writing, hunched over heavy oak desks inside cozy cottages in fragrant, peaceful pastures of Vermont. A memoir is written towards the end of one's life, too soon for me.

If Antoine had known that I have HIV, he might have understood why I felt experienced enough to write about my life. Previous dates with this man seemed awkward, so I hesitated to tell him—I didn't think we would become serious. We had dated only a few times, and I didn't feel much spark. Intense with little sense of humor, he telephoned me sporadically, usually at the last minute. Perhaps he thought me not mature enough, too silly. Maybe he was right.

In the movie *Little Big Man*, the grandfather character, Old Lodge Skins, decides that his life is over and declares to his family, "Today is a good day to die." Then he stoically walks away, closes his eyes and goes to sleep, he assumes forever. A few hours later he wakes up and asks, "Am I still in this world?"

"Yes, Grandfather," Little Big Man replies.

"I was afraid of that," he groans. "Well, sometimes the magic works, sometimes it does not." He looks a little embarrassed that he had miscalculated when he would die.

The grandfather was ready to die and like him I feel I have lain down, closed my eyes and waited to sleep—then die. But I too woke up and wondered, "Am I still in this world?" I am surprised to be alive writing this memoir.

Turning forty didn't seem bad. Fourteen years, and still well. Without disclosing the particulars, I told friends that I found forty a breeze. "Just wait," said one older friend, "fifty, that's the tough one." I have noticed that people who were upset when they hit forty had also fretted years before when they turned thirty. I have looked for clues to understand what personality types fret about aging, and which people take it in stride. A couple of my friends who are in their mid-sixties go out dancing together several nights a week and occasionally take classes to learn new dances. They are among the most graceful dancers on the Rock 'n' Bowl dance floor and many people, most of us younger, compete for a chance to dance with one of them. They seem to enjoy their lives as they take regular vacations to Honduras or Guatemala. They don't *appear* stressed out about age.

In my forties I find life better than I had dared to hope. I was not supposed to live this long. And I have stumbled across a subject that gives me an excuse to write a memoir. I have HIV, and at one time I thought I would soon die and would not have time to gain greater depth.

***

Antoine and I ran out of things to talk about. Without telling him that I had HIV, I could not tell him much about my memoir. And it was getting late, I was ready to go home. He walked outside with me towards my pickup truck, parked a couple of blocks away. We negotiated the cracked and buckled downtown sidewalks and passed by a voodoo shop where cool blue candles burned in the windows. Illuminated geckos raced up the glass, snapping at mosquitoes. I stepped through the warm steam of a grate-covered gutter and palmetto bugs scurried over the curb into the street. When we reached my car, Antoine gave me an awkward hug and said he'd call me. We both knew he wouldn't. I climbed into my truck, started the engine, and punched the radio button.

I thought about being forty years old, alive, driving this truck down the damp French Quarter streets of New Orleans. "The Soul Sister's Funk Show," was on WWOZ, the community radio station. Stevie Wonder's "Boogie On Reggae Woman" was just ending and Sly and the Family Stone's "If You Want Me to Stay" began playing. Sly's raspy, achy voice seemed to squeeze through the speakers. I was trying to figure out the secret to happiness as the vibrant horn section blew out bright stabs of sound. I turned up the volume, wishing I had a pair of those car speakers with the rumbling base that seems to hammer the air, and when I don't like the music, those speakers from a nearby car annoy me, but this was Sly and I wanted my truck to BOOM, BOOM, BOOM, BOOM. Sly sings,"*Because I promise I'll be gone for a while.*"

I turned it up and a wave of base rhythm filled my chest and I felt pretty sure that big speakers were the key to happiness.

I cruised down Rampart Street past clusters of people meandering towards the clubs: The Funky Butt, Snug Harbor, Café Brasil, Café Istanbul, Donna's and The Dragon's Den. A full moon painted slick streets with watercolor rhythms of light.

This memoir is about staying alive. I consider my survival an accident, and see life as random; yet I still try to understand why I live. As I write, as I think, as I stroll through the pungent, insomniac French Quarter or cruise highways through fogged-over swamps and bayous, a soundtrack shadows me and I imagine I will find clues encrypted in the rhythms or the melodies or the lyrics. I try to decipher the songs that keep playing in my jukebox head and I hope the music will send me a message.

On Weddings

THE PIZZA HAD JUST ARRIVED and Olan and I had planned an evening of watching videos. Olan paid the delivery boy and placed the pizza box on the living room table, then he pulled out of the front pocket of his jeans a delicate antique ring with a floral gold design detailed on each side of the band of tiny diamonds. At the time I was preparing to move to a new house and half-packed boxes sat stacked against the walls. Dust hung from the ceiling fan blades, piles of papers covered my desk and table, and the engagement ring rang softly in the center of the plum-walled room. I had heard of people with HIV marrying, but had not assumed this would happen to me.

For the wedding, I thought we had cooked up the perfect plan. Olan and I were flying to Brazil for two weeks to attend one of my Brazilian relative's Bar Mitzvah. I would fly from New Orleans and Olan would fly from Lafayette, near his home. We planned to meet in Miami, where, during an eight hour layover, we could take a taxi to the county clerk's office in Dade County, get married, eat a celebratory dinner at the nearest Pollo Tropical, taxi back to the airport, then fly to Brazil. Since we were flying to Brazil anyway, the honeymoon was planned Because I promise I'll be gone for a while we would just tack on a wedding at the beginning. We could be newlyweds in the streets of Salvador, Bahia; newlyweds dancing to Samba and Forro music; newlyweds stepping into very old Portuguese cathedrals, where beneath the layers of Catholic practices old Yoruba traditions stir like a repressed memory. And I could later tell my friends, "I had a Miami wedding," as if I had married in a tropical garden with bird of paradise flowers and banana trees and shiningly clothed bridesmaids. I wanted the promise of a future together but preferred to sidestep the hand calligraphed invitations. I wanted to step around the white lace bridesmaids, groomsmen in their rented tuxes, catered cakes and finger sandwiches, plastic champagne glasses and the guitar guy strumming love songs.

The way family members offered advice on how we should marry, I felt as though our relationship had become public property. I had not asked my family or friends which men I should socialize with. I did not ask who to date or with whom I should become intimate. I consider this private along with lifelong vows. I feared that if I had a wedding, I would feel detached, oblivious. The music, flowers, food and accommodations would be planned primarily for the pleasure of the guests rather than the guest(s) of honor, much like a funeral.

Olan is patient with my quirks. He assumed I would want a wedding, as this was my first marriage, his second. I think he was prepared to enjoy whatever sort of ceremony my parents and I cooked up. I begged Olan to let me bypass a public wedding and those sticky webs of etiquette. I hoped to slip away quietly. Perhaps Olan felt a little disappointed, but I find it hard to mask my boredom. I have become like one of those unselfconscious, smelly old biddies with wide-brimmed straw hat flopping over old-lady-blue hair as she walks down Magazine Street in lace-trimmed bobby socks. The older I grow, the less I care to please others.

I have participated in a few weddings. I was a bridesmaid at my sisters' weddings. In each case, I carried flowers and stood next to the bride. I don't remember much else except for my mom rubbing rouge into my cheeks, and a hair stylist curling my bangs, and bobby-pining clusters of daisies and baby's breath into my hair. I recall how guests held glasses of champagne in the air to toast the newlyweds.

***

My cousin Franklin drove Olan and me around Miami in his old, burgundy Oldsmobile. My heart pounded as sweat dampened the pink floral, crinkled rayon dress I had bought for this occasion. Olan looked handsome in his charcoal grey slacks and soft white embroidered shirt with a bolo tie hanging below the collar. The green stone matched his hazel eyes. I asked Franklin to drive faster but he cruised smoothly down 54th Street as we looked for signs pointing the way to the county clerk's office. We passed columns of palm trees and I tried to avoid looking at my watch, but I knew it was almost 4:00 p.m. and the office would soon close.

***

Maybe I'm still reacting to years of faking joy through my graduations and a confirmation. I dislike ceremonies, especially those in which I am expected to play a key role. My parents urged me to participate in my college graduation ceremony and although it didn't interest me, I complied. On graduation morning, I dressed, walked down to the auditorium, threw the robe over myself, and put on the mortarboard hat. I looked around and saw that the other graduates had dressed nicely; starched collars overlapped and good leather shoes and stockings peaked out from beneath the hems. My worn jeans and tennis shoes showed easily from beneath my robe. I had just thrown on the same kind of clothes I wore every morning. I thought the robe would cover me more completely, and my mind had been focused on packing to move out of the house I shared with two other students. The graduation seemed like something I just had to show up for. My mother later mused what a rebel I was—but this was not my intention. I was simply oblivious.

Franklin pulled into the left lane to turn onto 22nd Avenue where the office was located. We passed squat, bright green and pink-walled beauty parlors. I sang an altered version of the Dixie Cups song "Going to the Chapel."

> *Going to the DadeCountyclerk'soffice*
> *And we're gonna get ma-a-ar-ried*
> *Going to the DadeCountyclerk'soffice*
> *And we're gonna get ma-a-ar-ried*

I tried to sing high and girlie.

"You *sure* you want to marry her?" Franklin turned his head towards Olan in the back seat."

"I'm sure," Olan said. "I figure I'm being punished for some terrible deed I committed in a past life."

Franklin turned on the radio to drown me out and Stevie Wonder's "Boogie On Reggae Woman" was playing.

"Turn it up," I said.

"Gladly." Franklin reached for the volume control.

We pulled into the Caleb Center parking lot and saw numerous unmarked government buildings. I stepped out of the car by the curb and Olan and Franklin looked for parking. I rushed to the glass door of the County Clerk's office and pulled on the handle but it was locked. I saw a uniformed guard inside and I put my hands together to pantomime-plead, but he just shook his head and yelled, "Come back tomorrow!"

***

I first came to Grand Coteau, in Central Louisiana, during a year-long sabbatical. I rented a small house in a neighborhood filled with tall pecan trees and small, tin-roofed, wooden cottages with elderly people and families who made stews from the okra in their gardens and the squirrels they shot out of the trees. I intended my little house as a writing retreat. Olan and I met at Gram's, a neighborhood café, and eventually our paths began to cross regularly as I followed my two dogs, Tomboula and Samba, through the manicured lawns and wild pastures of the Jesuit college where Olan worked as Director of Maintenance. Tomboula and Samba plunged through blackberry briars after rabbits. Olan sometimes wandered with us and we watched eastern bluebirds scatter, saw downy woodpeckers swoosh between the tops of the live oaks.

***

After the Miami–Brazil layover wedding plans failed, I suggested several alternate venues and festivals: The Morgan City Shrimp and Petroleum Festival; the Louisiana Goat Festival; the Smoked Meats Festival; the Beaux Bridge Crawfish Festival; the Pontchatoula Strawberry Festival; the Zydeco Festival in Plaissance; the Washington Catfish Festival. I suggested we could sneak off to Gallup, New Mexico and get married on horseback. I asked him to consider the rich possibilities for the wedding announcements. "We are proud to announce our loping elopement on the slopes of Gallop!" But Olan said it would be trite to make our wedding plans based on word play.

**

I planned to tell Olan about my HIV status soon after we met so that if he was afraid, he would leave early, before I became fond of him. It was our second date, a warm evening, and though it was still light out, we heard owls calling from the arms of oaks in the field. Olan had cooked spaghetti for me in his home, a mobile home in the middle of a yellow-flowered field. I looked out the screen door and watched drowsy long-horn cows amble, trailed by snowy egrets. One brown and white patched bull chewed the leaves of a leaning sycamore tree. At the time I wasn't certain of Olan's level of interest in me, nor was I certain of my own. But in my past there had been occasions when I had underestimated a man's attraction to me, and by the time I revealed my HIV status, our relationship had become awkward.

Olan's dark curly hair had been cut and styled short, his ruddy face clean-shaven and he wore a pale green print shirt that matched his hazel eyes as we sat down to eat. "More spaghetti?" he asked, a waver in his voice. I could tell he had worried not only over the spaghetti but also about his appearance. He wanted to please, to make a good impression.

**

From the internet I pulled up a chart listing each of the United States' marriage requirements. According to this chart, twelve states require blood tests. About half of those states are in the South. Five states require a three-day waiting period, including Louisiana. In some states the waiting period can be waved by a judge. In some states, such as Florida and Louisiana, the waiting period is waved for out-of-towners, perhaps to attract "destination weddings," and to pump dollars into the local bridal industry. Olan and I considered marrying in Mississippi because it is next to Louisiana, so we could marry and honeymoon in just a weekend. But Mississippi requires a three-day waiting period. When I called the county clerk's office to inquire if this could be waived, I was told, "No, you'd probably have to go to Las Vegas for that." Maybe the rule stands to keep giddy, suddenly engaged couples of Sin City from seeping in over state lines.

***

Over brownies, I told Olan that I had HIV and I offered platonic friendship, trying to give him an easy out. I was surprised that this man from the country who had not met many people with HIV showed little surprise. He did not try to walk out the open door. In the first months of dating, Olan's eyes watched me and his words came carefully with his hopes that each outing would go right. He tried to anticipate which movies I might like to see, what I might like to eat and drink. He seemed more concerned with making a good impression than fears of HIV.

***

I was a bridesmaid at a good friend's wedding. Her mother bought fabric and gave it to us so that each bridesmaid could make her own dress to save money. At the time, I was trying to write research papers at the end of the college semester. So we hired a friend of my mom's, a skilled seamstress, to make the dress. I remember the dress was off-the-shoulder, to be worn with a strapless bra, a problem for my top-heavy figure. The spike heels left me unsteady and my friend kept asking me, "You'll be able to wear this dress again, won't you?"

I said no.

"Maybe at garden parties?" she suggested.

At the time I was planning a trip to Alaska to work on fishing boats. I realized that I had given the wrong answer.

"Yes, I'm *sure* I will wear this again," I said, trying to remember if I had ever been invited to a garden party. Each bridesmaid was told that when making our dresses, the hem should hang exactly twelve inches from the floor, not measured from the waist. Otherwise the dress hems would fall at slightly different levels which would look funny in wedding photos, we were told. Can't have all those hems doing their own thing, people would talk.

***

These days, I feel like a boat coasting from a shallow alcove into shifting seas. My mind passes between islands of short-term thinking and shores of long-term. I shift back and forth, trying to comprehend the nuances of living as an individual within a couple. I have lived alone most of my adult life. When I think of marriage vows, I stumble over "til' death do we part." In the past, perhaps it would have been an easier commitment for me because my life wasn't expected to last very long. But my life expectancy has expanded and now it's a life-long commitment that could last a real lifetime just like someone without HIV. Olan and I discuss life insurance and retirement, concepts I didn't used to believe applied to me.

***

I don't remember my parents suggesting what qualities to look for in a man when I was young, though they must have communicated something, as my boyfriends were usually kind, honest people. One memory that clings is the summer my parents enrolled me into a youth group at Schepps Jewish Community Center in hopes that I would make more Jewish friends. I was thirteen. Though we were not especially religious—we only attended Temple twice a year for the High Holy Days—I was told that I would only be allowed to date Jewish boys. I resentfully attended the youth group each week. In protest I brought a book to read rather than interacting with the other teens, my supposed future dates. When I eventually started dating, rarely did I date Jewish boys, despite my parents' protests. They had made the mistake of teaching me to accept people as individuals, regardless of ethnicity or religion, and this value seeped into my love life. In college, I did not mention my first serious boyfriend to my parents until I had gone out with him for about six months. He was a Chinese-American guy who played old Delta blues on guitar and complained that his parents pressured him to date only Chinese girls. I whined about my parents' expectations that I date Jewish boys; this was our first bond in a relationship that lasted for several years. My parents liked him and no longer mentioned their hopes that I would find someone Jewish.

***

I wanted to avoid blood tests as I already had blood drawn every three months, just before doctor's appointments. Out of curiosity, I called the Mississippi courthouse to find out what they would test for and I was told syphilis. Why syphilis, I wondered, as opposed to gonorrhea, chlamydia, herpes or HIV? I supposed this was an old law from when syphilis was a primary, incurable, sexually transmitted disease. Likely the requirement is intended to protect the infected individual and his or her partner as well as their future children. But I wondered what the public health office does if someone tests positive? Do they simply inform the individual and his or her fiancé? Do they counsel them on treatment? Does the information remain in the state records?   Medical records can be misused. Insurance companies could gain access to this information and choose to drop an individual's insurance.

***

A couple of my friends "snuck off" to Las Vegas for a quickie elopement. They stayed the weekend in a tacky, glitzy, red-velvet walled, casino hotel newlywed suite called "The Love Tub," for its heart-shaped Jacuzzi. I thought that sounded fun, and that they must have avoided offending anyone in particular, since no one was invited. But my friend warned me that you can still offend; she said that one branch of the family to this day feels certain that a public wedding took place but they were not invited! Another friend of mine eloped with her boyfriend during a cross-country bicycle trip. They later sent announcements with a photo of the two, arms wrapped around each other, paired bikes leaned up against a barb-wire fence. Behind them lay a soft green field, a bare damp road and above their heads a rainbow glowed against towers of grey rain clouds. I found the photo simple and romantic.

***

I wondered why I feel discreet about my relationship with Olan. In high school, I was careful not to mention to my parents the guys who I thought were cute. Though my folks encouraged me to have parties at the house with music and dancing, I pretended not to care. When asked out on my first date, I shyly told my parents about it. "Bye!" I called out as I tried to rush out the door, on my first date, to meet the young man who had just pulled up in the driveway in the yellow Trans Am he'd borrowed from his mother.

"No, you wait!" my mother said, insisting that he come inside so that they could meet him. He sat with us for a little while and talked with my parents. Later my parents and sisters said he was cute and often asked about him, though we only dated that one weekend. Although he was sweet and attentive, I found him unexpectedly clingy and I turned down his invitations to go out again. Maybe I am still inhabited by the shy girl who calls out "Bye!" as she rushes out the door.

***

The first item of community property Olan and I acquired was a travel account at the Hibernia Bank. Olan opened the bank account after we had been dating for about a year. At the time, I wondered if we would ever marry, as we sometimes discussed. I said that I loved to travel, even alone, and that I would not give it up for a relationship. Olan said that we could travel together, though the expense concerned him. I suggested that we open a joint bank account just for international travel, and we could each contribute $50 a month. After a year we would have $1200, enough to get us to Belize or Nova Scotia. After two years we might fly to Thailand, Cape Verde or Brazil. And if we did not dip into the account, after three years we could fly to Europe, the Middle East, Australia or Asia. As Olan sweated, ripping out rotten, mold-stench walls at work and I fretted over how to teach research documentation to restless freshmen, we could think about the day our bare feet would sink into the sand on a Portuguese shore where fishing boats haul in nets of fish for sale on the morning pier. Olan's eyes lit up. A month later he told me that he had opened an account and had deposited $100. We were investing in an amphibious, wheeled, winged sort of future; not the dead-weight, muck-sunk anchor sort of relationship I had feared.

***

Olan suggests we set money aside in case of an HIV emergency.

He does not say it, but I know he is thinking that if I became sick we will need the money for hospital expenses, lab work and medicines. "No," I say, unwilling to dwell on a disease that was predicted to kill me fifteen years before. I move between thoughts of an early death that does not come, and future years of retirement that once seemed unlikely. Am I growing old, or dying young? My aging friends, women who once took for granted their taut skin and bright eyes, fret over fading beauty. I, on the other hand, who once feared failing health, have become more confident of my vitality. We arrive from opposite directions and meet on this island of middle age.

***

I suspect that my parents hoped for a wedding even more because I am their youngest and because I have HIV. Perhaps in their minds my survival means that I hold the privilege of having a wedding and they have the privilege of watching me walk down an aisle holding a bouquet of pink and yellow roses, joined by the groom to say vows. But in my mind, survival means I can satisfy myself, even if my desires conflict with those of others. I insist on the right to skip the ceremony and elope in a busy airport with our minds and bodies ready to fly. Sometimes when I speak to my mother on the phone, I feel tension buzzing like a fruit fly trapped inside the telephone lines.

***

There's a certain cry I hear in songs that gets me, that pulls me into the spin of the sound. You can hear it in the whine of Townes Van Zandt, Al Green, Lucinda Williams. It's like a water spirit emerging from the well of the throat. That yodel-cry that rises up in sounds of country, zydeco and folk—think Willie Nelson, Boozoo Chavis, Bob Dylan—and the sound tastes salty like ocean, pungent like swamp water. A slap-in-the-face stench assaults your nostrils and awakens your senses; the whiny yodel-cry may sink deep into the pit of your stomach. Sometimes I feel like pain affirms life more than joy does. Or maybe the pain and beauty contrast. I may be the sort of person who would take life for granted were it not for the remembered stabs of the first time a needle slid into my vein

141

to draw blood to track changes in my t-cell levels. Memories needle me and fear sometimes rises up like that blues cry. The sweet voice carries an edge, a tremble of uncertainty; it cracks and gives character to the music that follows the heartbeat base.

***

The second piece of community property Olan and I acquired was a 10-foot, flat-bottom boat. It came as a surprise when we were visiting a couple of friends in Grand Coteau. That afternoon we sat beneath the trees petting our hot-breathed dogs and pushing away dragonflies that tried to light on our glasses of beer. My friends planned to give the boat away and asked if we might like to have it. By the time the case of beer was finished off, we had a boat and a trailer with which to tow it. In my mind, we had a vehicle that could take us through the cypress groves of the Atchfalaya swamp lands. Olan and I could eat chicken sandwiches while we watched alligators propel through the bayou. Great blue herons would lift up from the cypress branches and climb through the air.

***

Olan and I eloped one long weekend at the Galveston County courthouse. And we keep saving for our next travels and to buy a motor for our boat. We will glide through the Atchafalaya basin, find passage through the grasses and groves of trees. Early morning breezes brush against our necks. A water bug skates the water surface until it disappears into the well-mouth of a fish that descends back down below. I sing to Olan all of the water, fishing, and pond songs I can recall, usually remembering only one or two verses; songs about fishing, swimming, drowning, leaving the water, returning to the water, sinking into a well. I think of Al Green's "Take me to the River," John Prine's "Fishin' In Heaven," Taj Mahal's " Fishin' Blues," Nick Drake's "River Man." I think of being afloat in the boat listening to crows' throaty calls. I don't know how to end this story because I cannot see the end. Olan and I roam the waters hungrily.

***

I have written a book about what does not happen.

My life is like this: the zydeco accordion player plays on and the set continues. One song rambles on, the notes draw out that bluesy sound and finally the long song ends, the musicians leave the stage and you figure the set has ended.

It is way past midnight on the bar's neon clock.

The musicians will soon pack up their bags and go home, the stage will clear, the dance floor will empty, but the guys over there in the corner still smoke their cigarettes, flirting with the women. Saxophones, guitars, the base, accordion and rubboard lie askew on the stage. It is time for everyone to go home, but the players in their jeans and boots and cowboy hats drink beer in the parking lot. It must be time for them to go home.

Nothing happens.

Then, boots step back onto the stage. This is just a long break as the music again begins to build and the dancers return to the floor as this life continues a bit longer. Those dancers out there on the floor are not thinking about the end of the set; their lives are normal, but all of our lives are normal and mortal. I put money in the tip jar as the band plays on. All the dancers shove dollars into the tip jar as a gambler feeds coins into a slot machine.

And drunks slide quarters into a jukebox to draw out the voices of Patsy Cline, Lyle Lovett, Townes Van Zandt, Willie Nelson, Nathan and the Zydeco Cha Chas.

Voices wail from the car radio, howl from the neon lit jukebox in the corner, those voices call inside my head and remind me that I live.

Po-Boy Contraband

ACKNOWLEDGEMENTS

A heartfelt thanks goes out to the following publications in which portions of this book previously appeared.

Turning Up the Volume (Xavier Press, 2005).
"Mid-City Rock 'n' Bowl." *New Orleans: What can't be Lost* (UL Press, 2010).
"My Movie," *52%*. The Womyn's Centre, Ottawa, Ontario. Spring, 2002.
"HIV Survey," *HEArt* (Human Equity Through Art). Spring, 2002.
"Intimacy," *ACORN*. Spring, 2002.
"Rearranging the Furniture," *Prism International*. Spring, 2001.

_____

I give my thanks to the many who have encouraged and supported me, and those who shared the stories with me.

I appreciate the Wurlitzer Foundation who granted me two tranquil Fellowships in the Mountains of Taos New Mexico. I also give thanks to Creative Capital's Professional Development program and the Louisiana Office of Cultural Development/Division of the Arts for including and inspiring me through Creative Capital's "Strategic Planning" retreat. Thanks to Olan for understanding my need for solitary time, and for helping me to transform an Acadian cook house into a writing studio.

More thanks to:

• Xavier University Press and Thomas Bonner for publishing *Turning Up the Volume* in which many of these essays first appeared
• Amy Clipp for offering her insightful feedback in the early stages of this project
• to the Owl Writing Group for offering encouragement in the last stages of this project
• to my parents and sisters for support and encouragement
• to friends and family members for patience and tolerance as they were transformed into characters for the purposes of these essays
• to Ken Waldman for his example of unshakeable determination,

and for introducing me to my publisher, J.L. Powers
• To J.L. Powers for her wise, editorial comments

Some of these essays are intimate and raw. I hope this book brings music to your ears, rhythm to your life, and hope into your heart.

If you feel sorrow for me, please express your sympathy through gifts of high quality dark chocolate—Dutch or Swiss is preferred.

A Note On the Cover Image

The image of the winged figure on the cover was created by Louisiana artist Kelly R Guidry.

Guidry was born and raised in Lafayette, Louisiana. His mother is a seamstress specializing in elaborate Mardi Gras costumes, and her parents were also artistically inclined. His grandfather worked in cast metal while his grandmother created large scale, intricate works using braided fiber. At a young age, Guidry showed his artistic inclination, preferring to draw or create small things rather than play sports.

But it wasn't until college that Guidry discovered not only his artistic medium—sculpture—but that he preferred to use a chainsaw rather than a mallet and a chisel. An instructor taught him welding and pushed him to develop his own rough edged style that Guidry calls "Modern Primitive." He uses modern technology to execute concepts inspired by the artwork of primitive cultures.

Though he majored in advertising and worked at an ad agency for a few years after graduating, he soon realized he had to stop pretending—he needed to embrace art fully.

For more information about Guidry and his artwork, please go to his website, www.kellyguidry.com.

CPSIA information can be obtained at www.ICGtesting.com
Printed in the USA
LVOW12s0547101013

356307LV00001B/19/P